KU-763-392

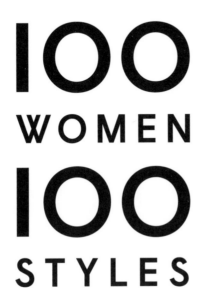

LAURENCE KING

Published by
Laurence King Publishing Ltd
361–373 City Road
London EC1V 1LR
United Kingdom
Tel: +44 20 7841 6900
www.laurenceking.com

A catalogue record for this book is available
from the British Library

ISBN: 978-1-78627-485-4

Picture research: Giulia Hetherington
Design: Mariana Sameiro
Printed in China

Laurence King Publishing is committed to ethical and
sustainable production. We are proud participants in
The Book Chain Project ® bookchainproject.com

BOOK CHAIN PROJECT

Front cover: Twiggy, 1967 (Paul Popper/Popperfoto/
Getty Images)
Back cover: Audrey Hepburn, c.1954 (Hans Gerber/
ETH-Bibliothek Zürich/Com_X-H061-002/CC BY-SA 4.0)

100 WOMEN 100 STYLES

THE WOMEN WHO CHANGED THE WAY WE LOOK

TAMSIN BLANCHARD

CONTENTS

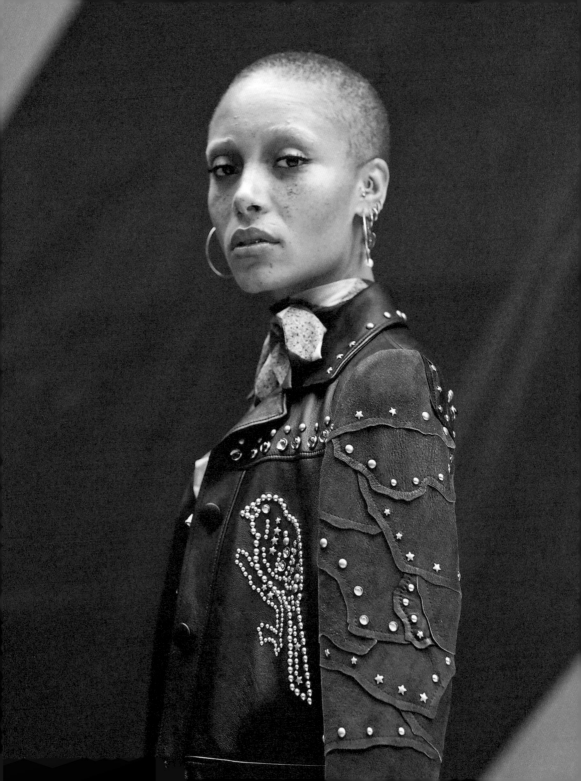

INTRODUCTION

Putting together a list of 100 women who have changed the way we look was easier than you might think. Don't we all already have a list of women whose style we admire, or who have influenced the clothes we wear, the shade of lipstick we choose, the way we style our hair? These women electrify us when we listen to their music, watch their films or read about their pioneering work, and then stay in our memory banks forever as subliminal guides. There will be differences in all our lists, of course, yet there are some women who rise above generational divides, whose distinctive spirits and styles are constantly inspiring.

There are the stars of the silver screen: Marilyn Monroe, whose glamour captivated in *Some Like It Hot* (1959); Lauren Bacall, whose cool demeanour was irresistible in those timeless black-and-white films that are always worth a watch; Audrey Hepburn with her neat gamine polo necks and ballet pumps in 1957's *Funny Face*, the film that introduced countless viewers to the fabulous world of the fashion magazine (long before *The Devil Wears Prada*). Then, of course, there's Winona Ryder with her leather jackets and wayward individualism, an instant cult star after her role in the ultimate mean girls' movie *Heathers* (1988).

In 1984, Madonna burst on to our TV screens like a rush of adrenaline, with a bare midriff and a jangle of plastic earrings, singing 'Holiday'. It was a time of sartorial daredevilry in music, as women appeared on our screens flaunting a unique image that was almost more important than the music: Siouxsie Sioux's aggressive Cleopatra brows, Kate Bush's wild hair and Lycra leotards and Poly Styrene's bonkers Oxfam-chic. The world of sophisticated jazz singers also offers inspiration: just look at Billie Holiday with her signature white gardenia; Sade Adu and her long, sleek plait, hoop earrings and red lips; and Amy Winehouse, her overblown beehive decorated with cocktail umbrellas and a brightly coloured scarf.

The fashion industry not only provides idols of impeccable style and taste but also of fierce independence, who, refreshingly, refuse to play by the rules – think Coco Chanel, Rei Kawakubo, Vivienne Westwood.

These 100 women have broken the rules, worn the trousers, burnt the bras and then worn them proudly in an empowered expression of their sexuality. By forging their own paths, our style sisters have given us the freedom to express ourselves however we choose.

This book, then, is a celebration of those who have caught our eyes, given us food for thought and, many times, stopped us in our tracks.

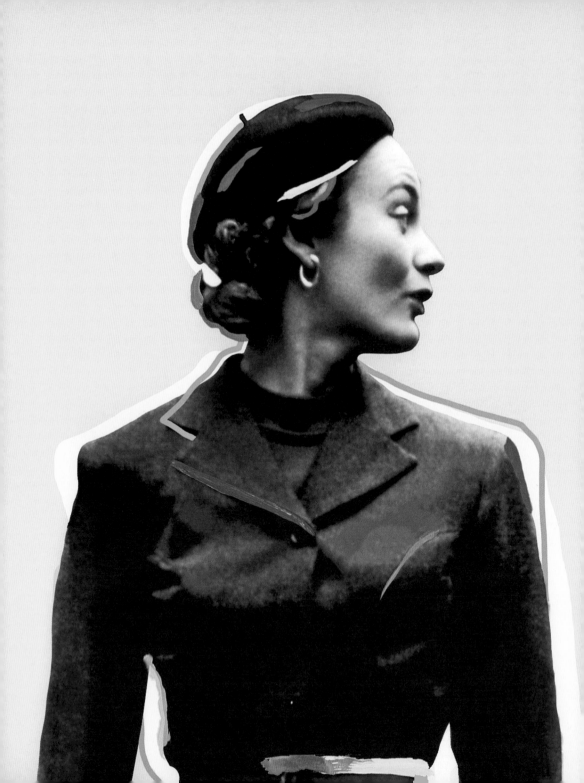

Fashion Plates

These are the women who have crystallized the look of a given moment and channelled the direction of fashion in their own particular way. Much more than just pretty faces, these women have influence, poise, personality, their own perspective and, it goes without saying, an endless sense of style.

LISA FONSSAGRIVES

Sweden, 1911–1992

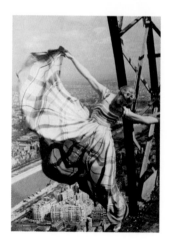

When Erwin Blumenfeld photographed Lisa Fonssagrives hanging effortlessly from the Eiffel Tower, her skirt billowing in the wind, Paris was on the brink of war. It was May 1939, and the world, like Fonssagrives herself, seemed to be on the edge of a precipice.

A decade later Fonssagrives had become a household name, the original supermodel. She was the first model to be on the cover of *Time* magazine, with the line: 'Lisa Fonssagrives: Do illusions also sell refrigerators?' The magazine described her as 'a billion-dollar baby with a billion-dollar smile and a billion-dollar sales book in her billion-dollar hand'.

In 1950 Fonssagrives married the photographer Irving Penn, and together they created real magic. She was 39, but her experience, intelligence, poise and absolute control complemented his austere photographic studies perfectly. Whatever she wore, whether a Balenciaga coat fit for a duchess or a witty black-and-white harlequin coat for a ball, she understood how to wear it with ultimate panache. She would carefully choreograph every element of the image, from her pose and her facial expression to the folds of the fabric and the position of her elegantly shod foot.

What made Fonssagrives so successful was not just her aristocratic nose and her cheekbones, but the way she treated modelling as a craft. She would look at an outfit in the mirror, studying the way the light fell on it, and how to pose and move in it to do it justice. She had been a dancer and a student of art and sculpture, and she brought a strongly visual sense to her work. When she did her first test with *Vogue Paris*'s most famous photographer, Horst P. Horst, she visited the Louvre Museum to study how women wore clothes in paintings, what they did with their hands, how they turned their heads.

Although she downplayed her role, Fonssagrives elevated the status of the model to be at the core of the creative process, resulting in intense moments between herself, the clothes she was wearing and the photographer's lens. And when model and photographer are so closely in tune, the result is timeless perfection.

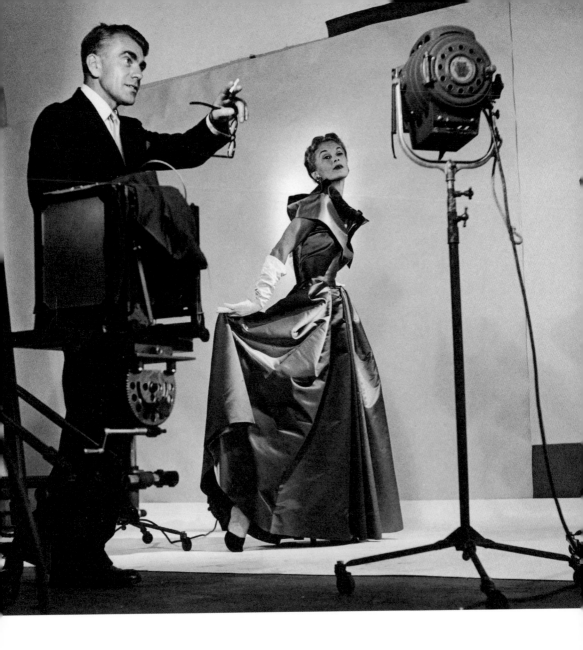

'It is always the dress, it is never, never
the girl. I'm just a good clothes hanger.'

DOVIMA

USA, 1927–1990

'I would just never appear in public without looking like Dovima, who was to me an image of myself.'

Dovima hailed from a time when haute couture reigned as the wardrobe for the elite, and fashion was the realm of grand women, aristocrats and heiresses who all seemed to know one another. With her haughty, glacial look that hinted at money, good breeding and a lavish lifestyle, she personified the archness and grandeur of 1950s Paris.

But while she may have looked like the epitome of mature, upper-crust, untouchable fashion, the reality was anything but: Dovima was the child of a Polish-American policeman and an Irish woman, and was brought up in Queens, New York. Scouted in 1949 by a fashion editor at *Vogue*, she was being photographed by Irving Penn the following day. Conscious of the tooth she had chipped as a child, she adopted an enigmatic, demure smile that resulted in her being compared to Leonardo's *Mona Lisa*.

Dovima had natural poise, whether she was looking down her nose as she stepped out in a grand Jacques Fath gown or holding hands with a monkey while dressed in Givenchy. Such was her success that she was the first model to be known by just one name (a combination of her three first names, Dorothy, Virginia and Margaret); she was also known as the 'Dollar-a-Minute Girl'.

The relationship between Dovima and the photographer Richard Avedon was magical. His photograph of her standing regally between two extraordinary elephants at the Cirque d'Hiver in Paris in 1955 is historic. Her arms are gracefully posed, her body a perfect, streamlined curve in a black velvet dress with a silk sash – the first to be designed by a young Yves Saint Laurent for his mentor, Christian Dior. 'She was the last of the elegant, aristocratic beauties,' Avedon said, calling her 'the most remarkable and unconventional beauty of her time'.

Dovima stopped modelling as 1960 heralded youth and a looser, more democratic fashion, and overnight she looked as though she belonged to another age. Tragically, she ended up working as a hostess at the Two Guys Pizza parlour in Fort Lauderdale, Florida. An original print of the photograph with the elephants sold for $375,000 at Sotheby's in April 2018, an eternal snapshot of a fleeting fantasy.

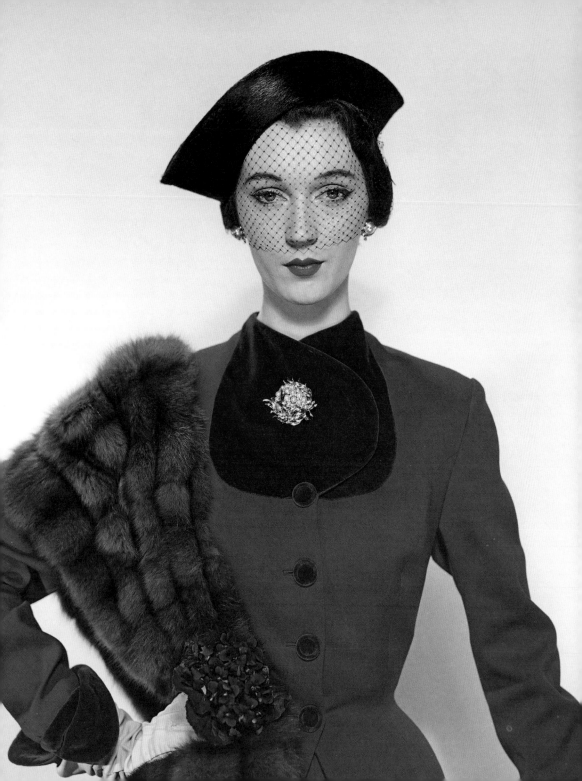

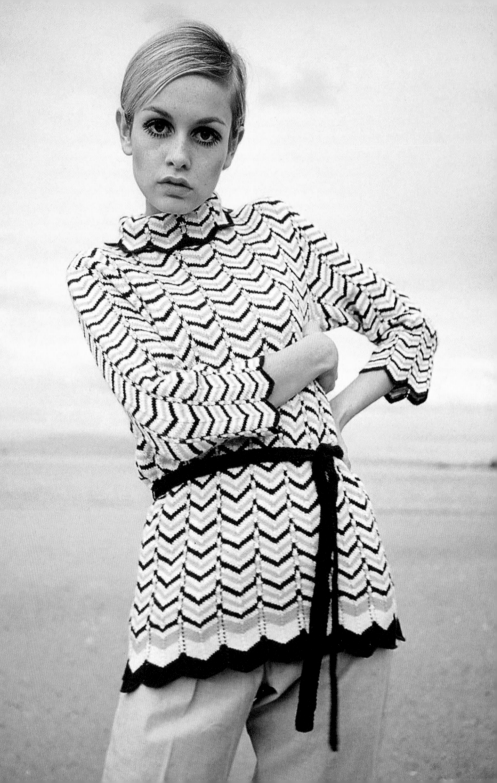

TWIGGY

UK, born 1949

'I came to represent not just that one decade but the whole free-wheeling, free-loving, free-thinking Sixties revolution.'

When the *Daily Express* ran a double-page spread of Twiggy with the headline 'I Name this Girl the Face of '66', Lesley Hornby was just a 15-year-old schoolgirl. She was short for a model – just 1.7 m (5 ft 6 in) – and straight up and down like a stick. Her boyfriend's brother had called her Twigs.

Twiggy was already a regular at Biba, the revolutionary new department store selling cool fashions that she could actually afford. She loved clothes and made her own, and had already decided that she wanted to go to art school to learn fashion design. Not tall enough to be a fashion model, she managed to get a contract doing beauty shots and was sent to the celebrity hairdresser Leonard. He gave her a radically new, short haircut that turned out so well that he had her photographed. With her long neck, neat head, big eyes and drawn-on bottom eyelashes, she looked startlingly new. Twiggy was born.

For the first time, it was possible for a working-class girl from north London to become a world-renowned model. Before Twiggy, most star models – including her idol Jean Shrimpton – were from aristocratic or wealthy backgrounds, filling time before finding a husband. For Twiggy, modelling was a career, a chance to see the world, meet amazing people and be financially independent.

When she first went to New York, in 1967, Twiggy and Justin de Villeneuve, her 25-year-old worldly-wise boyfriend and manager, were met with Beatles-like mania. Swinging London was seen as the coolest place on Earth, and Twiggy was symbolic of a new era in fashion and female independence. She was a pioneer for a new generation of teenagers who were discovering their own voice and style, setting the stage for the innocent youthfulness of Kate Moss and the play-acting of Cara Delevingne, both of whom never really took modelling, their own beauty or the fashion business that seriously.

In 1971 Twiggy starred in the 1920s-style film *The Boyfriend*, and began to focus on becoming a stage actor. Twiggy-mania had lasted only four and a half years, during which time extraordinary images by photographers including Richard Avedon and Bert Stern had captured a unique spirit who will inspire generations to come.

PENELOPE TREE

UK, born 1949

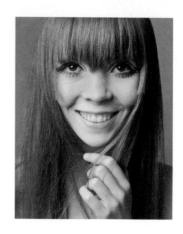

*'People thought I was a freak.
I kind of liked that.'*

Penelope Tree's alien beauty – huge, cartoon-like eyes, impossibly long arms and legs, incredibly fine features – perfectly suited the mood of the late 1960s, and fashion designers such as Pierre Cardin, who were inspired by space travel and an optimistic vision of the future. She looked as though she had just stepped off a flying saucer.

Tree's mother, a socialite, worked at the United Nations and had little time for her as she grew up. She was sent to the UN School, a fact that explains her precocious knowledge of the world. In an interview with Polly Devlin in *Vogue* in 1967, the 17-year-old's conversation ranges from Rasputin and modern poetry to the films of W.C. Fields and Dorothy Parker's Round Table. And, of course, make-up. 'Eventually, I'll end up like a layer cake or a Zulu war mask,' she joked. She started wearing it at the age of 13, creating a different look each day, and even shaved off her eyebrows. She enjoyed getting a reaction from her friends' parents (her own were rarely around).

Tree had the sort of privileged, wealthy upbringing that gets you spotted by Diana Vreeland (see page 36) at Truman Capote's star-studded Black and White Ball in New York in 1966, and transported straight to the pages of *Vogue*. 'She projects the spirit of the hour,' wrote Devlin, 'a walking fantasy, an elongated, exaggeratedly huge-eyed beautiful doodle drawn by a wistful couturier searching for the ideal girl.'

As the spirit of the hour, Tree helped to define – and influence – the look of the late 1960s. Her six-year affair with the photographer David Bailey sealed her position as It girl supreme, from sleek mod to barefoot hippy in a miniskirt decorated with fox tails. But in fact she was anything but in control of her life. She was too young, too thin (she suffered from eating disorders) and, after she developed a skin condition that left her unable to model, cast aside by the industry that celebrated everything that made her so vulnerable.

It is troubling now to perpetuate Tree's influence on fashion, rooted as it was in such an unhealthy, impossible body image. But at the time such topics were not discussed so freely. It is positive to reflect that times change and that, even at the height of her fame, she was considered an extreme and other-worldly ideal of beauty.

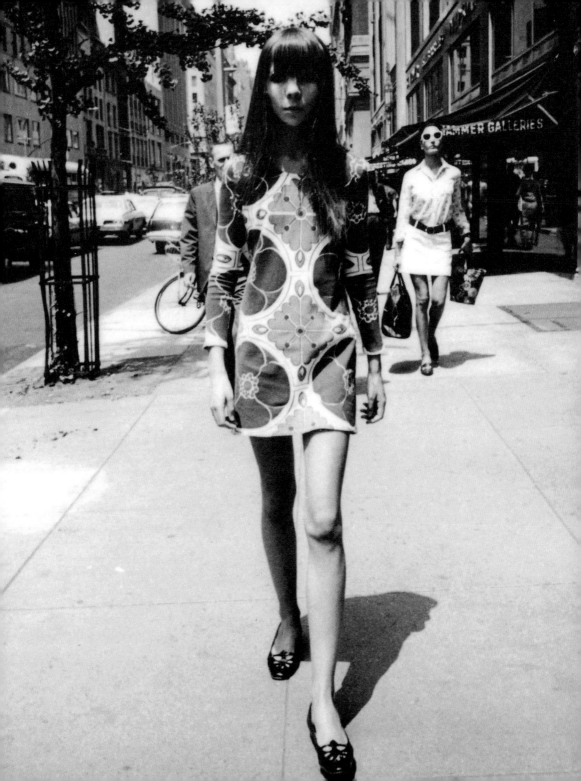

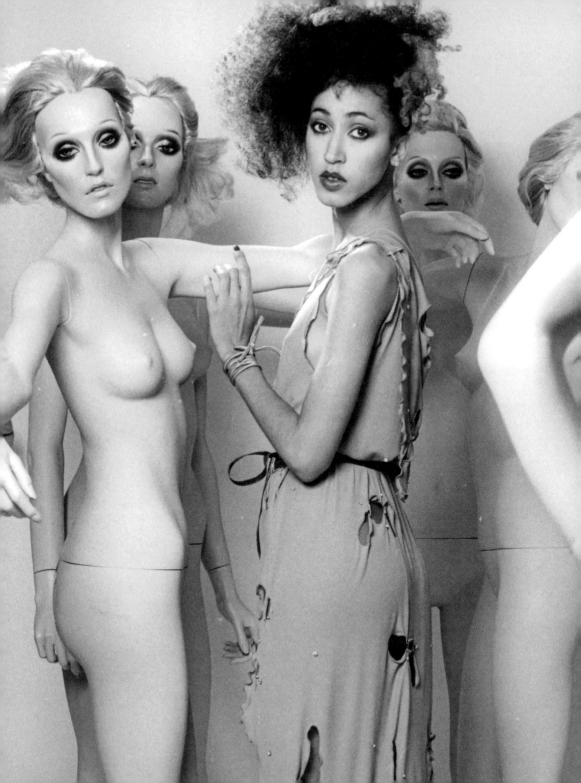

PAT CLEVELAND

USA, born 1950

'I looked at the magazines and I didn't see anybody who looked like me.'

Friends with Andy Warhol and Karl Lagerfeld, Pat Cleveland was one of the fashion illustrator Antonio Lopez's legendary 'girls', the group that also included Jerry Hall, Jessica Lange and Grace Jones – fashion's coolest gang in Paris in the early 1970s. Her twirling, dancing, energetic appearances on the catwalk were the perfect reflection of the disco-dancing, hyperactive, optimistic, liberated spirit of that pre-AIDS era.

Cleveland grew up in Harlem in a poor but creative household with her mother, Lady Bird Cleveland, a single parent and artist. At school Pat, who was part Cherokee, part African American, part Irish and part Swedish, never fitted in: 'I was too light to be black, too black to be white and too skinny to be pretty.' When she was 15, she was spotted on the subway by Carrie Donovan, an editor at *Vogue*. Donovan liked her outfit – a miniskirt (before anyone else was wearing them) and a houndstooth hat she'd made herself – and the magazine ran a story on her as a young design talent before calling her back to model the latest looks. Cleveland also caught the eye of the Ebony Fashion Fair and started modelling Paris couture looks as part of its all-black-model roadshow.

Told that she would not make it as a photographic model because there simply wasn't the market for 'girls like her', Cleveland left for Paris, where she became a muse for Lopez, who was illustrating the pages of *Vogue* and Andy Warhol's *Interview*. Her circle of friends included Lagerfeld, Valentino, Yves Saint Laurent and even Salvador Dalí. In 1974, when Beverly Johnson became the first black woman to be featured on the cover of *Vogue*, Cleveland returned to a more inclusive, freewheeling New York. There, she became a regular at Studio 54 and friends with the designers Halston and Stephen Burrows.

Cleveland had her own unique, urban streetwise style. Designers would give her clothes to wear because she made them look so cool. With her mass of curly hair, she helped to create the disco glamour look of the 1970s, laughing and dancing her way down the catwalks. In her sixties she continues to model, often with her daughter Anna Cleveland, who has followed in her twirling, high-heeled footsteps.

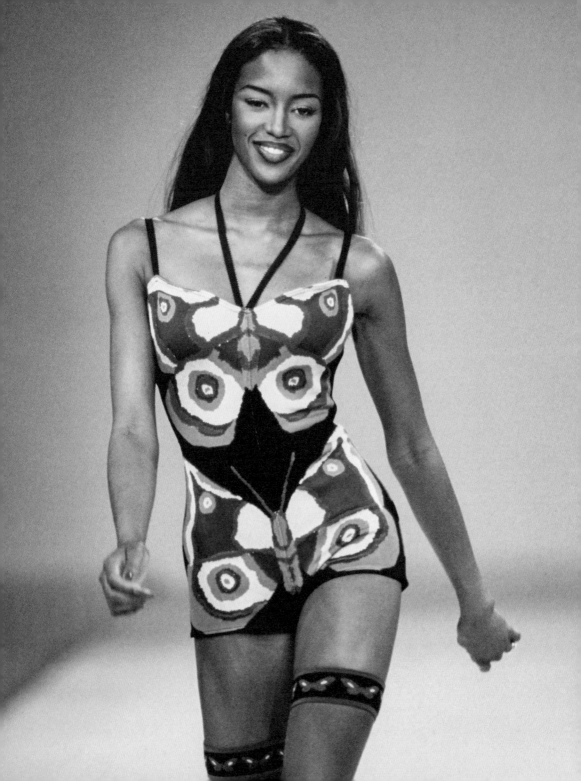

NAOMI CAMPBELL

UK, born 1970

'I make a lot of money and I'm worth every cent.'

It was not *Vogue* that made Naomi Campbell a cover girl, but the new British magazine on the block, *Elle*. In April 1986 the seventh issue of the magazine heralded a new attitude to fashion for a fresh generation of intelligent young women. Campbell was 15 when Martin Brading photographed her for the cover. She looked fresh-faced and unbelievably pretty, her hair cut into a messy bob (I remember taking my copy to the hairdresser and asking for the same cut). She looked approachable but very cool, the personification of that Levi's 501s and Dr. Martens fashion moment.

Campbell was one of the holy trinity of supermodels, alongside Linda Evangelista and Christy Turlington, with a distinctive sashay that made her a catwalk superstar. After taking her under his wing when she was just 16, the fashion designer Azzedine Alaïa became her surrogate godfather (she called him 'papa' and he called her *'ma fille'*). In December 1987 she was on the cover of British *Vogue*; the ultimate accolade followed in 1989, when Anna Wintour put her on the September cover of American *Vogue*.

The current editor of British *Vogue*, Campbell's long-standing friend Edward Enninful, is inspired by her personal style, which he has described as 'a touch of India, a touch of seventies, a touch of beachy sexy; mix in a vintage fur. We take what she normally wears and amp it up.' She started out as a young gazelle of a schoolgirl and is now one of the most experienced figures in the world of fashion and publishing. In 2017 she appeared on the catwalk for Donatella Versace with the other original supermodels, on the twentieth anniversary of Gianni Versace's death.

Campbell continues to model, but, in her new role as a contributing editor to British *Vogue*, she now has the power to bring positive change to the industry that also shaped her, particularly when it comes to diversity. In 2013 she formed the Diversity Coalition with fellow models Iman and Bethann Hardison. Given the Fashion Icon award at the Council of Fashion Designers of America's Fashion Awards in New York in 2018, Campbell said: 'I stand here today as a proud woman of colour, and I will continue to push for diversity and equality in this industry.'

KATE MOSS

UK, born 1974

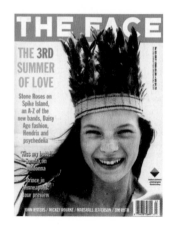

'Never complain. Never explain.'

In the beginning it was about her youth, her precious adolescence, her teenage disregard for adult rules and regulations. Kate Moss had that 'so what?' look in her eyes, with the cheekiest grin that was both innocent and rebellious.

At just 1.7 m (5 ft 6 in) tall, Moss had to be exceptional even to find work as a model, let alone become the face of a decade. But the 1990s were all hers. Rather than stacking shelves in a Croydon supermarket, she found herself on the cover of *The Face* magazine, topless on Camber Sands, wearing a a feather headdress. That cover from 1989 signifies the beginning of a new era in music and fashion. In November 1992 Marc Jacobs showed his infamous 'Grunge' collection for Perry Ellis, and Moss was the star of the show. She was 18, wearing the sort of clothes on the catwalk – sloppy T-shirt, beanie, tartan skirt and Dr. Martens boots – that she would be happy to wear on a day off. The next month Moss appeared on the cover of *Harper's Bazaar*, photographed in New York. A contract with Calvin Klein followed, and her face soon became recognized around the world.

Throughout her career, and with a string of rock 'n' roll boyfriends including Johnny Depp, Pete Doherty, Jamie Hince and Jefferson Hack (the father of her daughter), Moss has always retained an air of cool – and of privacy. She has never felt obliged to justify or explain her behaviour, whether it has to do with her weight, her smoking or her drugs bust. She has inspired designers from Marc Jacobs to John Galliano and Alexander McQueen, who created a haunting 'Pepper's Ghost' hologram of her for his 'Widows of Culloden' show in 2006. The ghostly, flickering figure was re-created in 2011 for the exhibition 'Savage Beauty' at the Metropolitan Museum of Art in New York and the Victoria and Albert Museum in London.

When Topshop asked Moss to design a collection in 2007, crowds queued to buy their own piece of Moss magic. Designing a collection was easy: she simply looked through her own wardrobe and picked out her favourite pieces – slip dresses, biker jackets, waistcoats and trouser suits. When Edward Enninful became the editor of British *Vogue* in 2017, he made Moss a contributing editor. It was a no-brainer. For 30 years she hasn't missed a beat, and her fashion barometer is not likely to fail now.

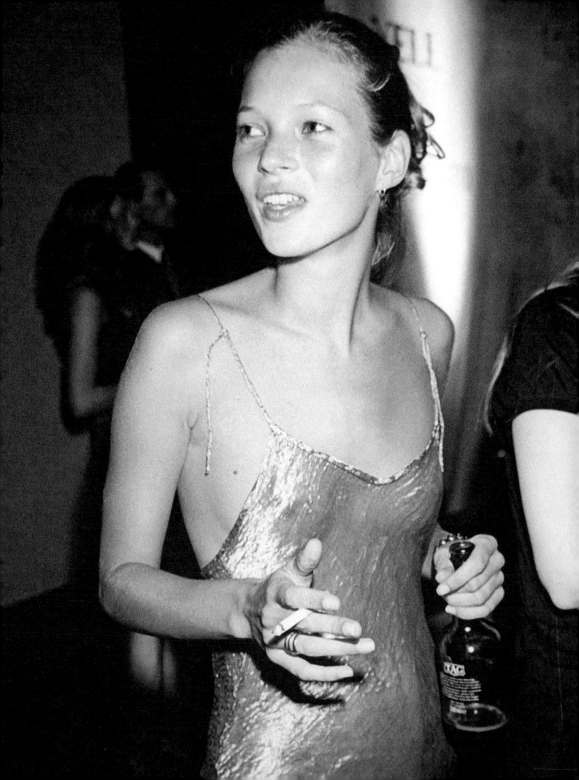

ADWOA ABOAH

UK, born 1992

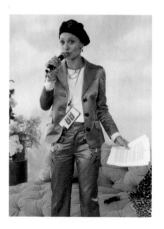

Adwoa Aboah is one of the first models to have used her visibility and platform as a model to talk about some of her demons, including depression and drug addiction. She speaks to a new generation of young women who have been given the chance to talk about anxiety, mental-health problems or even how to deal with rejection – something that models rarely discuss but must deal with daily.

Aboah's platform, Gurls Talk, exists both online (www.gurlstalk.com) and as a series of events to encourage girls like her to share how they are feeling. She has talked about her self-hatred and isolation as a teenager, and the lack of support available to her at school. 'I wanted to be like all the other girls. Blonde. White, blue eyed,' she has said, revealing that she wore a hat for two years because she was ashamed of her hair. At the age of 14, in an attempt to numb her emotions, she became addicted to the tranquillizer ketamine and was sent for treatment. She then attempted to commit suicide by overdosing, but managed to find a more positive path after spending time in rehab.

As a highly successful model – the glamorous cover girl for Edward Enninful's first issue of British *Vogue* – Aboah is in a profession that is all about appearance and superficiality. But she is opening a path for a wider understanding of beauty. From her lowest days of self-hatred – of not wanting to be herself – she has grown into a poised and brave speaker who uses her voice to help other girls and young women find the light at the end of the tunnel. Aware of a responsibility to provide the help she needed at school but didn't have, she is trying to open the doors to the fashion and modelling industry to women and girls of all demographics, shapes and sizes.

Out of all her achievements, Aboah is most proud of the work she does with Gurls Talk. The secret to finding confidence and success as a model, she says, is 'not being embarrassed on set. No one cares, no one's judging, just do your thing.' And Aboah's thing is about as cool as it gets.

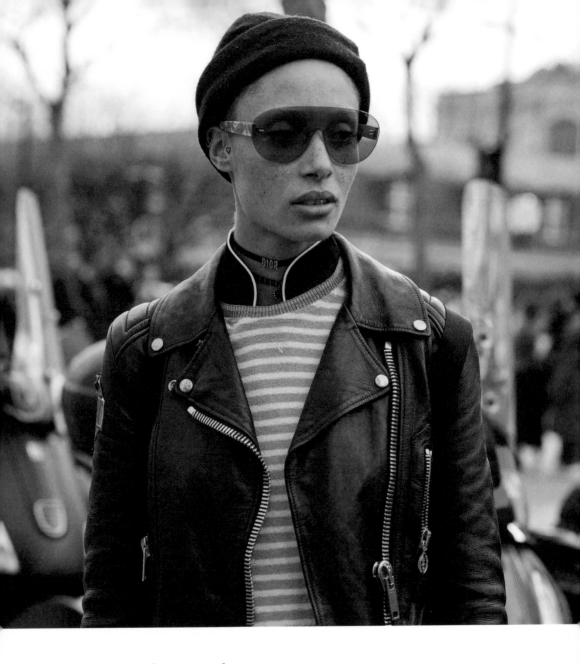

'It's about who you are as a person,
and what you stand for.'

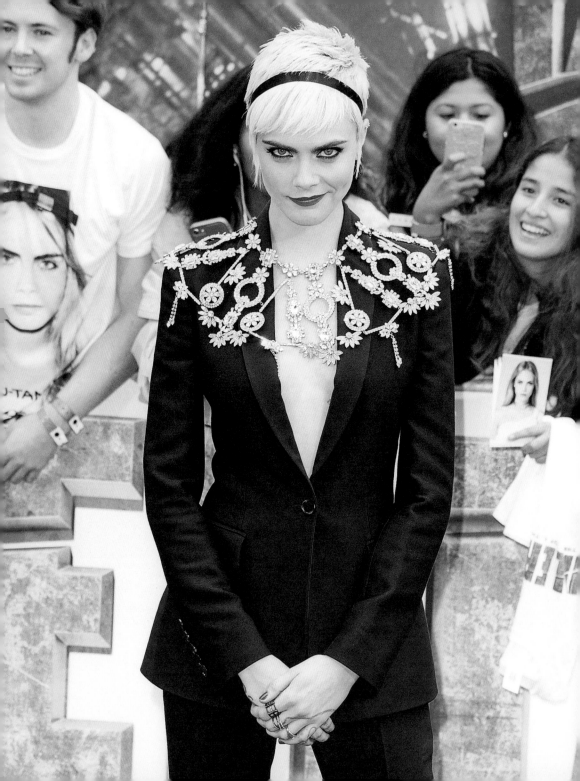

CARA DELEVINGNE

UK, born 1992

'Embrace your weirdness.'

You can't help loving Cara Delevingne. She is extraordinarily beautiful, but seems to have a complete disregard for life as a high-flying fashion model. The tattoo on the bottom of her foot declares that she is 'Made in England', a reference to the way modelling made her feel as though she was an inanimate object.

The fashion world that Delevingne just about tolerates adores her for being herself. It loves her honesty, although at times it is bemused by her cross-eyed twerking, her bed head, her fondness for an animal onesie and her ironic sportswear. Karl Lagerfeld has declared her the 'modern It girl'. And then there are the eyebrows, which have a life all their own. According to the *Guardian*, Delevingne's thick, unruly brows will define the decade as Twiggy's eyelashes did the 1960s: 'It is thanks to Delevingne – or Her Eyebrowness … – that young women everywhere now have a brow icon.'

Delevingne's difficult relationship with modelling has been superseded by the career in acting that was always her dream. In 2015 she was perfectly cast as the dark and disturbed Margo Roth Spiegelman in an adaptation of John Green's 2008 cult novel *Paper Towns*. She has also started out as a writer: her Young Adult novel *Mirror, Mirror* (2017) is about a girl who, like her, vents her excess energy and frustration on a drum kit. She has spoken out about the depression she suffered as a teenager, her mother's heroin addiction and her irritation at the beauty industry's narrow-minded definition of beauty, and is open about her bisexuality.

In 2015 Stella McCartney told *Vogue*: 'The thing about Cara is that she's more than just a model – she stands for something in her generation's eyes. She has a fearlessness about projecting what she stands for, which is so rare.' Delevingne is the woman who refuses to follow rules, a social-media superstar (as Green said, she's 'good at the internet') who has discovered that her voice is her most effective weapon. We are never sure what she will do next, but we do feel that there's no holding her back – with Delevingne, almost anything is possible.

GIGI HADID

USA, born 1995

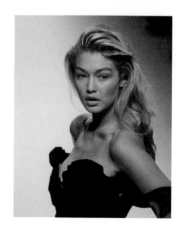

'My personal motto is "Eat clean to stay fit, have a burger to stay sane."'

With more than 41 million followers on Instagram at the time of writing, Gigi Hadid is a social-media phenomenon. She has more power than most publishing houses, giving her unparalleled influence over everything from the clothes we wear to the shade of lipstick we buy. She can make – or break – a brand with a single Instagram post, and is part of a new breed of entrepreneurial Instagirls who use social media to fuel their million-dollar careers. She has total control of her image, her brand endorsements and the way she communicates with her followers. It's hard work being Instagram-famous. Her short-lived split from her boyfriend Zayn Malik was made official not via a statement to the press but by the singer unfollowing Gigi and her mother on Instagram.

With her younger siblings, Bella and Anwar – who also model – Hadid has changed the way designers work with models. When she collaborates with a designer such as Tommy Hilfiger, it is an equal partnership. She not only wears the clothes for advertising campaigns, but also is the named designer for a capsule collection. She has single-handedly revived the Hilfiger brand for a new generation, and there is a Gigi x Tommy Barbie doll to prove it.

Hadid, who has a Palestinian father and a Dutch reality TV-star mother, is not the typical size zero catwalk model, and is proudly curvaceous. Her weight fluctuates because of Hashimoto's disease (an autoimmune condition affecting the thyroid gland), but she says she doesn't diet and is partial to a bacon cheeseburger and the odd gingerbread cookie. In 2016 she was named International Model of the Year at the British Fashion Awards by Donatella Versace, with whom she also collaborates as a photographer.

With power comes great responsibility. Hadid has spoken out about representation in fashion (after *Vogue Italia* retouched an image to make her skin look three shades darker than it actually is), but her power to change things for the better was harnessed in June 2018, when she announced that she was working with UNICEF. She tries to stay grounded, and has said: 'My mum always told me if you're not the nicest, most hard-working girl in the room there's always going to be someone prettier than you who's nicer and more hard-working.'

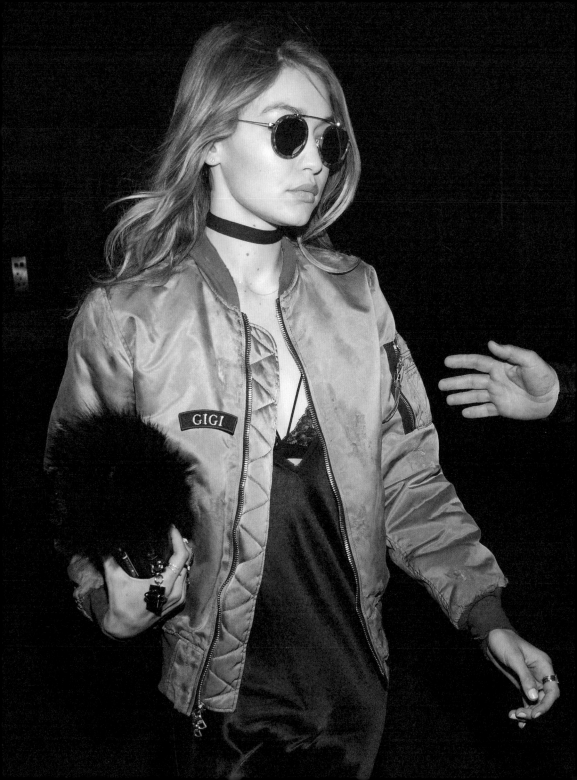

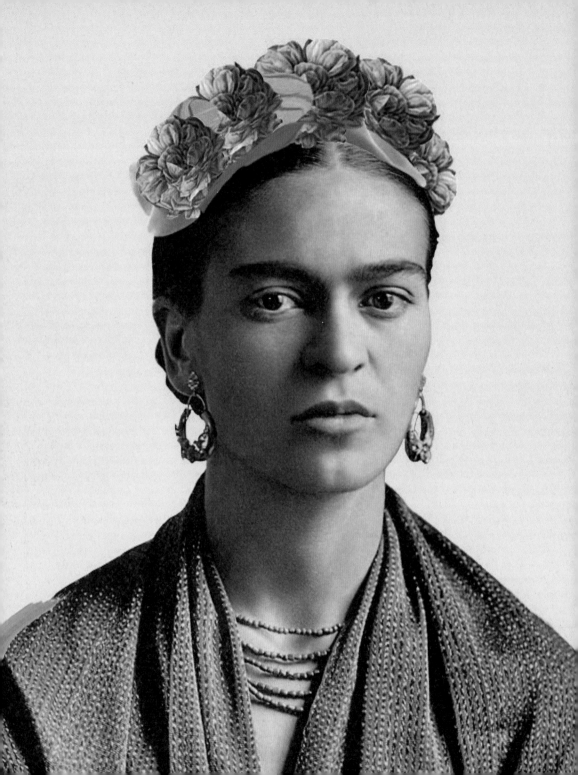

True
Originals

Women who have their own distinctive
style tend to be enormously strong as
individuals. Or is it the other way around?
Either way, they create their own style,
whether it's a carefully honed uniform
or an ever-changing parade of dazzling
peacockery; they never follow fashion.
True originals refuse to be pigeonholed
or defined by anyone or anything. They
are their own women.

LUISA CASATI

Italy, 1881–1957

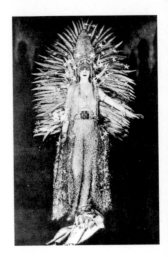

'I want to be a living work of art.'

You couldn't make Marchesa Luisa Casati up if you tried. Imagine a woman who wore a dress made of light bulbs (it short-circuited, giving her an electric shock); who turned herself into a human fountain made of pearls and wire; who dyed her flame-red hair green for a party so that it matched the colour of the flames when iron filings were thrown into a fire; who kept a boa constrictor as a pet, along with a jewel-collared cheetah, a clutch of white peacocks and her beloved greyhounds.

Casati was a decadent figure, 1.8 m (6 ft) tall and rake-thin. At night she would float around the canals of Venice on a gondola, naked under her fur, her face powdered deathly white, her eyes apparently sinking into their sockets under the weight of her false eyelashes and kohl, or she would host seances to make contact with the dead. She was a bit of a monster – casually poisoning her servants with toxic gold body paint when she used them as extras for parties – but she was adored by the artists, sculptors, designers and poets who she generously supported.

Unspeakably rich, Casati spent the fortune she had inherited from her father on hosting the wildest parties and making herself the centre of the art and fashion scene. It was the stuff of opium-fed dreams. One dress was constructed from a net of glittering diamonds, surrounded by a sun of gold feathers, to represent light. She might complete an outfit with a necklace of snakes, or dress her hair with white peacock feathers and dribble chicken blood down her arms. An obsessive exhibitionist, she shocked polite society out of its wits and set the taste for her times – if you dared to keep up with her.

No wonder Casati is the source of never-ending inspiration for designers, including John Galliano (for his first Dior couture show in 1998), Alexander McQueen, Karl Lagerfeld and Dries Van Noten – all of whom have dedicated entire collections to her. Chanel even located its cruise collection for 2010 at the Venice Lido, one of Casati's favourite stamping grounds, creating pared-back dresses and coats in iridescent gold and silver, long and narrow, just like the Marchesa, and a make-up palette inspired by her green eyes. Casati's enduring influence on the fashion world – Georgina Chapman named her ill-fated Marchesa label after her – is so pervasive that elements of her style can be seen everywhere, from peacock prints to the subtle drape of a wrap, the fullness of a sleeve or the fine pleats of a dress.

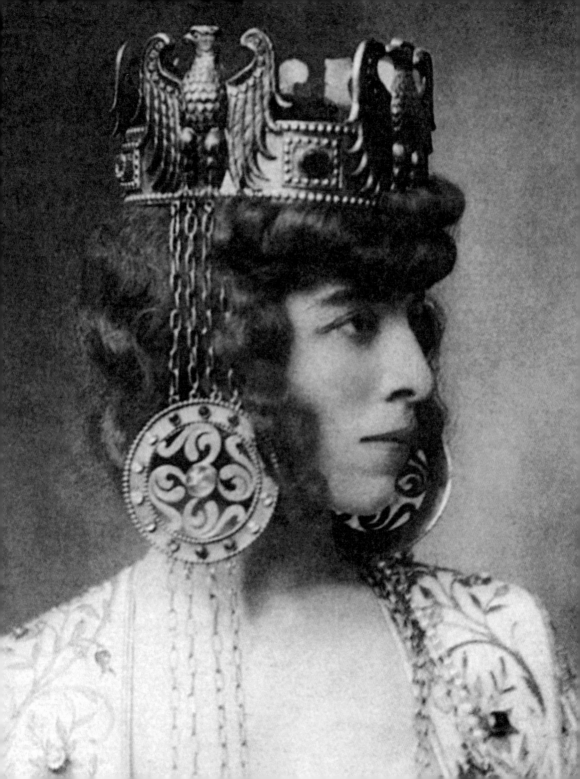

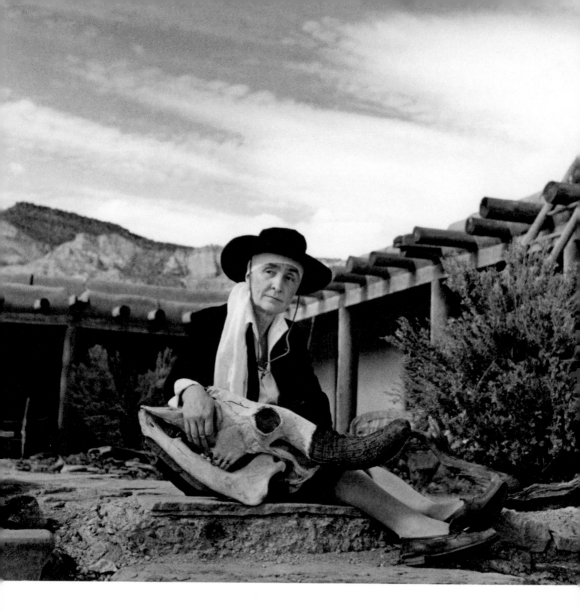

'I've been absolutely terrified every
moment of my life and I've never
let it keep me from doing a single
thing that I wanted to do.'

GEORGIA O'KEEFFE

USA, 1887–1986

Georgia O'Keeffe was a true bohemian, a pioneer and a puritan with a touch of the cowboy both in the way she wore her jeans and in her love of the great outdoors, which inspired her work. Looking at her scrubbed face, sack-like dresses and flat shoes, you might be misled into thinking photographs taken of her in the 1920s are from the present. Her life and her androgynous mid-century modernist American style have both been well documented, not least by her husband, the pioneering photographer Alfred Stieglitz, who took some 330 images of her as an ongoing portrait.

Known as the 'mother of American Modernism', O'Keeffe was the first female artist to be given a retrospective at the Museum of Modern Art in New York, in 1946. Some 70 years later a show at Tate Modern in London combined her paintings, photographs of the artist and some of her clothes, including her kimono collection; her embroidered blouses and bolero jackets, some of which she made herself; her timeless wrap dresses; her well-worn flat shoes; and a man's three-piece suit that she ordered at the age of 93.

At first O'Keeffe split her time between New York and New Mexico, where she went on solitary six-month painting trips, but she set up home permanently in New Mexico in 1946, after Stieglitz died. She wore her Levi's with deep turn-ups because they were more practical that way when she was riding her motorbike (an image that has inspired many fashion shoots), accompanied by men's shirts. She wore few accessories or superfluous decoration, and preferred simple, pared-down shapes. Dior's creative director Maria Grazia Chiuri used O'Keeffe as the inspiration for her cruise collection for 2018.

Bruce Weber took the final portrait of O'Keeffe in 1984, when she was 97. She chose to wear a black Japanese kimono, her signature *vaquero* hat and a much-loved brooch, a present from its maker, the artist Alexander Calder. Even at the end of her life, art, life, nature and style were inseparable for her.

DIANA VREELAND

France, 1903–1989

'Style – all who have it share one thing: originality.'

Think of the archetypal eccentric fashion editor and you will picture Diana Vreeland. Everything she did was larger than life. If it wasn't extraordinary, it wasn't worth doing. She said that 'too much taste can be boring', which brilliantly sums up her own style that always made you look twice. It might be the red patent knee-high boots with an otherwise sober black outfit, the excessive number of Verdura bangles piled on her arm, her penchant for wearing one colour, particularly red, head to toe (often to match a room setting), or simply the way her lacquered red fingernails matched her lips so perfectly. She was a true original, and for her, clothes were a form of theatrical entertainment.

Vreeland began her career in fashion in the late 1930s after being spotted dancing in a Chanel dress by Carmel Snow, the editor of *Harper's Bazaar*. Vreeland had always loved clothes, and used *kabuki*-style make-up – white powder, red lips and rouged cheeks – to enhance her striking, unconventionally strong features. The helmet of lacquered black hair, Japanese warrior-style, came later. Her ability to think creatively about fashion resulted in a regular column in *Harper's Bazaar*, 'Why Don't You …', a list of camp, witty, outlandish suggestions for thinking differently about what you were wearing. Her ideas included nifty little tips such as tying tulle bows to your wrists or turning an old ermine coat into a bathrobe.

Vreeland joined *Vogue* in 1962 and became editor-in-chief the following year. Richard Avedon described her as 'the only genius editor' of the magazine. All that mattered to her was the final image. Budget or basic practicalities were never a consideration. She had an incredible eye and absorbed historical, cultural and pop references like a sponge.

Such was Vreeland's renown that she was the inspiration for the editor Maggie Prescott in the film *Funny Face* (1957), and for the avant-garde Miss Maxwell in William Klein's film *Who Are You, Polly Maggoo?* (1966).

Vreeland was always a step ahead of the pack, and could see a trend before anyone else did. Her spirit of adventure and no-limits imagination and curiosity still inspire many of fashion's most original and creative minds today.

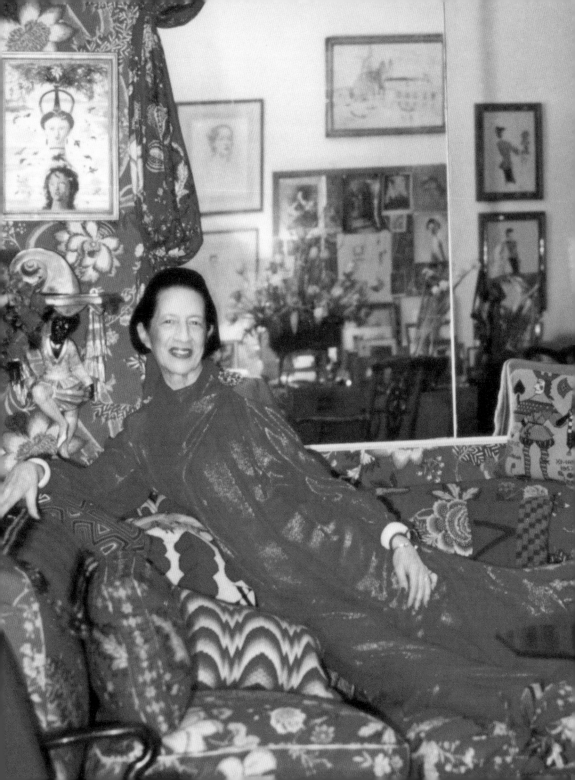

FRIDA KAHLO

Mexico, 1907–1954

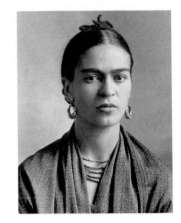

'*I never paint dreams or nightmares. I paint my own reality.*'

If Frida Kahlo were alive today, she would be the selfie queen, the influencer of influencers. It is easy to imagine her spearheading the Women's Marches against Donald Trump – the hashtag #monobrow would be her badge of honour. But she didn't do too badly when she was alive. Of her 143 paintings, 55 are self-portraits, the first painted in 1926, when she was confined in a body cast after an accident on a bus in Mexico City.

Through sheer determination Kahlo managed to walk again, and continued with her painting. She became caught up with the muralist Diego Rivera and his world of artists, photographers, bohemians and communists. Despite his inability to keep his hands off other women, he and Kahlo were married in 1929; she was 22 and he 42. They lived in separate houses built next to each other, and it was a tempestuous, unconventional relationship. Kahlo herself had many affairs, some with women, and one, in 1937, with Leon Trotsky.

Kahlo's most famous painting, *The Broken Column* (1944), depicts her body held together by a corset and nails, her spinal column crumbling inside her. Despite her pain and suffering, it is her joyful, colourful style that has captured people's imaginations and made her an inspiration to countless fashion designers, from Jean Paul Gaultier to Stefano Gabbana and Domenico Dolce. She is said to have started wearing the traditional long Mexican skirts to cover her limp after suffering polio in childhood. For such a tortured soul, she was a riot of colour and decoration, her hair piled up in braids wrapped with bright scarves and fabric and embellished with flowers. The embroidered Mayan *huipil* blouses she wore were handwoven, each one unique.

Kahlo used her clothes to emphasize her Mexican Indian roots and her national identity. Her clothes were discovered in 2004, sealed up in her house on her husband's orders until 50 years after her death. In 2018 they formed part of a major exhibition dedicated to Kahlo at the Victoria and Albert Museum in London, inspiring a new generation to discover the strength, beauty and vivacious style of this magical artist.

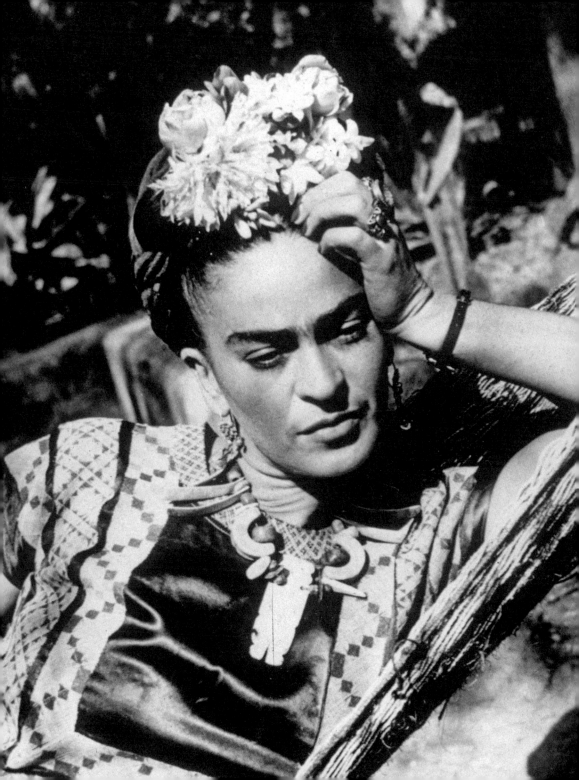

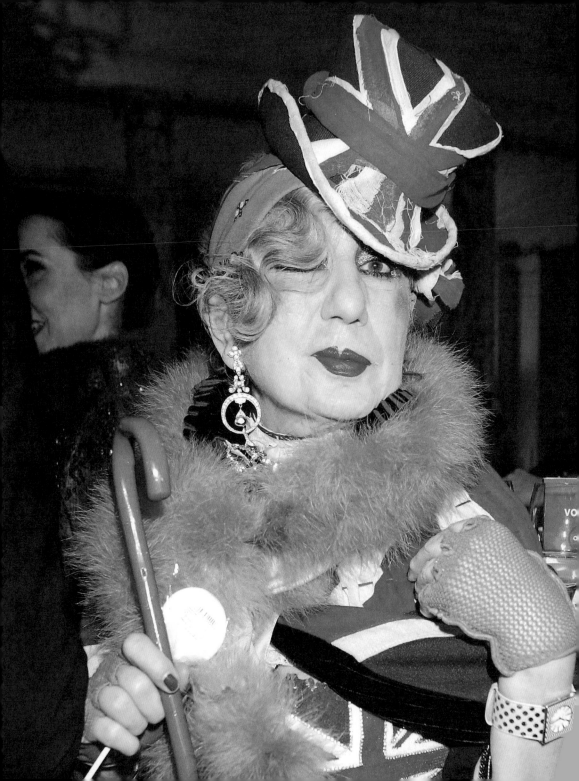

ANNA PIAGGI

Italy, 1931–2012

'My philosophy of fashion
is humour, jokes and games.
I make my own rules.'

Anna Piaggi was a walking work of art. Each outfit was a collage, a mix of periods, fabrics, old and new, luxury and throwaway (although she never did throw anything away), high and low, serious and funny. She had no boundaries and followed no rules. She saw getting dressed in the morning as an opportunity to express herself as an artist might with a few strokes of paint. She might wear what appeared to be a fruit bowl on her head, a stars-and-stripes scarf at her neck and a couture gown, and finish it all off with a red plastic cane.

Born in Milan, Piaggi started working as a translator for a press agency in the 1950s. There she met her future husband, the photographer Alfa Castaldi, who became her lifelong creative collaborator. In 1962 she became the fashion editor of *Arianne* magazine and began travelling regularly to London, where she frequented her friend Vernon Lambert's stall at Chelsea Antiques Market, buying up pieces of clothing that she would both research and wear. 'I have dresses that should be in museums that only cost me $50,' she said. However rare and valuable, she wore them all.

From the early 1980s, Piaggi was never seen without a hat, and she enjoyed a lifelong friendship with her co-conspirator the milliner Stephen Jones. She also loved to play with make-up, powdering her face like a Venetian mask, her Cupid's-bow lips precisely painted, her eyes ringed in dark kohl, her eyebrows carefully arched and kiss curls highlighted the perfect shade of blue.

Piaggi was a collector of clothes as well as of ideas and images. For an exhibition at the Victoria and Albert Museum in London in 2006, she lent some of her extraordinary collection of 265 pairs of shoes, 29 fans, 932 hats, 2,865 dresses, 24 aprons and 31 feather boas. The clothes she collected from antique stalls and flea markets formed the inspiration for her monthly column 'Double Pages' for *Vogue Italia*. This was made up of scrapbook pages filled with illustrations (which she loved), notes, thoughts and observations – a reflection of whatever was capturing her imagination.

Manolo Blahnik described Piaggi as 'modern beyond belief', and Karl Lagerfeld loved to draw her. She was a constant source of inspiration, and her frivolous imagination and creativity were manifested in whatever she wore. She cultivated a new way of talking about fashion and opened the door for people to experiment and play with their clothes.

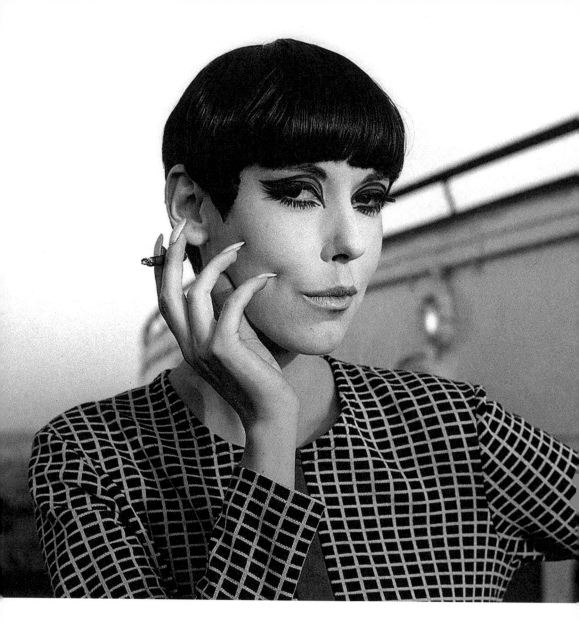

'I used to change the way I walked by what
I wore. If it was a little girl dress, I might
walk pigeon-toed or I would often spoof
it ... I liked to have fun with clothes.'

PEGGY MOFFITT

USA, born 1940

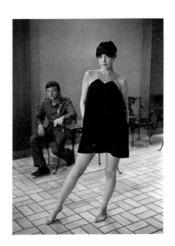

'She was born with well-cut hair and doll's eyes.' So begins *Pretty Pretty Peggy Moffitt,* a picture book by the children's writer William Pène du Bois, who dedicated the book to the model in 1968, at the height of her fame. He drew her wearing fashion designs by her friend Rudi Gernreich.

It was as Gernreich's controversial model that Peggy Moffitt rose to celebrity. One image in particular, published in *Womens Wear Daily* in 1964, was a defining image of the 1960s: Moffitt is bare-breasted, wearing the designer's monokini, complete with her super-sharp Vidal Sassoon five-point bob and big, doll-like panda eyes. It was taken by Moffitt's husband, William Claxton, who was better known for his photographs of jazz musicians and Hollywood stars. The monokini was, for Gernreich, a protest against sexual repression. He believed in fashion as a way of making social commentary and creating change in society, and Moffitt was the perfect conduit. In 1967 they made one of the first fashion videos together, *Basic Black,* directed by Claxton.

Moffitt's long, lanky body, cap of razor-sharp hair, eyelashes, expressive features and whole way of moving – she never seemed to sit still, and always appeared to be dancing to some fabulous soundtrack all of her own – was as crucial to the 1960s as Mary Quant's miniskirt (see page 84). Moffitt was the ultimate gangly girl, partly feminine, partly masculine, comfortable in her skin, straddling the worlds of fashion and art and joyfully unselfconscious about it. When she was cast for a scene in the William Klein fashion film *Who Are You, Polly Maggoo?* (1966), she became the blueprint for all the other models, who were all styled to look like her. She wasn't just ultra-modern, she was the future.

In 2006 the Chicago rock band the Handcuffs released the album *Model for a Revolution* with an image of Moffitt on the cover. 'Peggy Moffit, you're an inspiration, original, not the imitation', they sang. And she was an original, the most extreme version of herself that she could be.

REI
KAWAKUBO

Japan, born 1942

*'I find beauty in the unfinished
and the random.'*

Nobody looks at fashion the way Rei Kawakubo does. Her trademark bob and head-to-toe black outfits, often finished with a beaten-up leather jacket, have remained unchanged over the years, as has her uncompromising vision of what she believes to be fashion. That vision, however, can be strange, unsettling, unlike anything you have seen before. And that, of course, is why she is the fashion world's original spirit.

Kawakubo is not influenced by the things that influence other designers – their travels to exotic places, their visits to art shows, things they see in magazines, the work of other designers. Her ideas appear to come from a more abstract place. She thinks in terms of silhouettes, structures, positive and negative space, the duality of life, rather than traditional notions of dress. The harder it is to understand, the more successful the collection. If someone questioned the wearability of one of her looks, she would say they had missed the point.

In 2017 Kawakubo's label Comme des Garçons was the subject of an exhibition at the Metropolitan Museum of Art in New York. 'Rei Kawakubo/Comme des Garçons: Art of the In-between' showed 140 pieces by Comme des Garçons, from the ripped and shredded collections that shocked Paris in the early 1980s to the abstract sculptural creations of the present day. Typically, it was touch and go whether Kawakubo would attend the opening gala night thrown in her honour (her clothes may be extrovert, but she prefers to stay behind the scenes); in the end she did appear, wearing a white leather biker jacket with a voluminous black skirt made from a mound of origami folds, a pair of black trainers and what appeared to be a piece of white string in place of a tiara around her geometric haircut.

Kawakubo is often referred to as the designers' designer, and admired for her radical, rule-breaking approach to fashion. One of her biggest achievements has been to make black the colour of the fashion pack. She is also an incredible businesswoman, and has made her world accessible to anyone who can afford one of her cult fragrances or a T-shirt from her phenomenally popular brand Play.

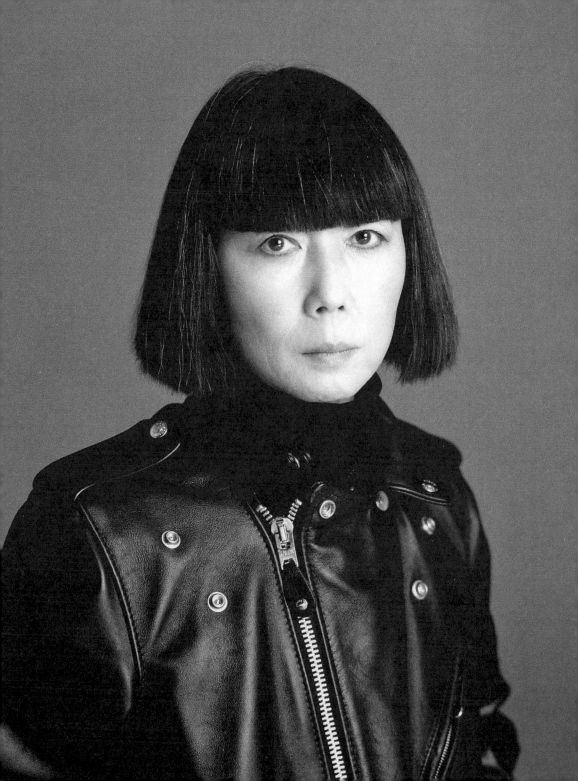

TINA CHOW

USA, 1950–1992

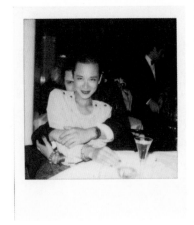

*'You have either to bring beauty
or ugliness ... and you're not
allowed to bring ugliness.'*

According to Karl Lagerfeld, Tina Chow invented minimalist chic. She had perfect taste, and with her short, sleek Eton crop, anything she wore – whether a pair of Kenzo jodhpurs or an Armani jacket – looked effortlessly cool.

Chow started out as a model, and her American and Japanese heritage made her and her sister, Adelle Lutz, highly sought-after as models in Japan. As Tina Lutz she was the most famous model there in the 1960s, and had a contract with the beauty brand Shiseido. After her marriage to the ultra-fashionable restaurant entrepreneur and art collector Michael Chow, she took on a new role as society queen and hostess in London. Mr Chow was the epicentre of the city's fashion and art scene in the 1970s; when it opened in Knightsbridge in 1968, the Rolling Stones and the Beatles were there. It was that sort of place. As muse to many an artist and designer, including Andy Warhol, Yves Saint Laurent and Lagerfeld,

Chow would welcome everyone from the illustrator Antonio Lopez to Warhol, David Hockney, Keith Haring and Jean-Michel Basquiat. Nobody went to Mr Chow for the food: with her wardrobe of vintage Fortuny clothes and vintage pieces from flea markets, Tina was the star attraction.

In the mid-1980s, having lost many friends to AIDS, Tina Chow devoted more and more time to working with AIDS charities, and when she was herself diagnosed as HIV positive, she talked openly about her disease, becoming the first high-profile woman to do so. After her death, an exhibition of Chow's fine collection of twentieth-century costume went on show at the Fashion Institute of Technology in New York. It included pieces by Paul Poiret, Romeo Gigli and Azzedine Alaïa, and some choice examples of Balenciaga and Fortuny. 'Tina had an innate elegance and never needed any designer to do anything for her,' said Giorgio Armani. 'Rather she did a lot for us.'

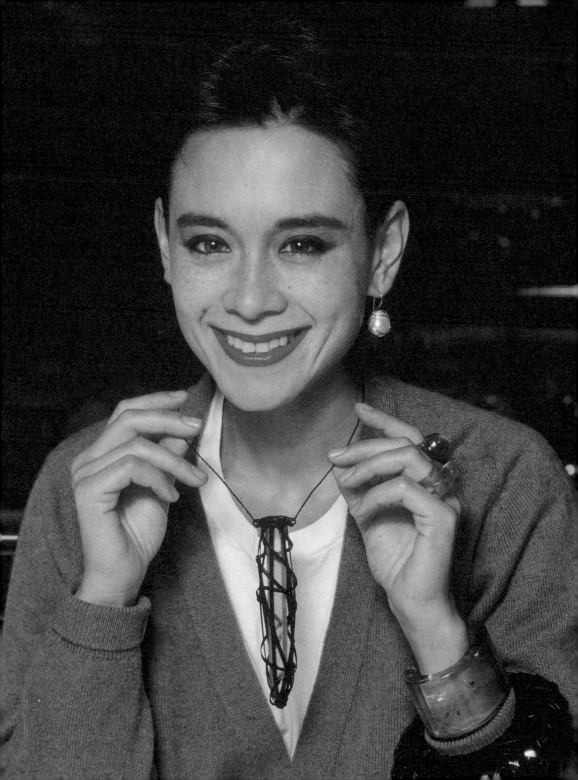

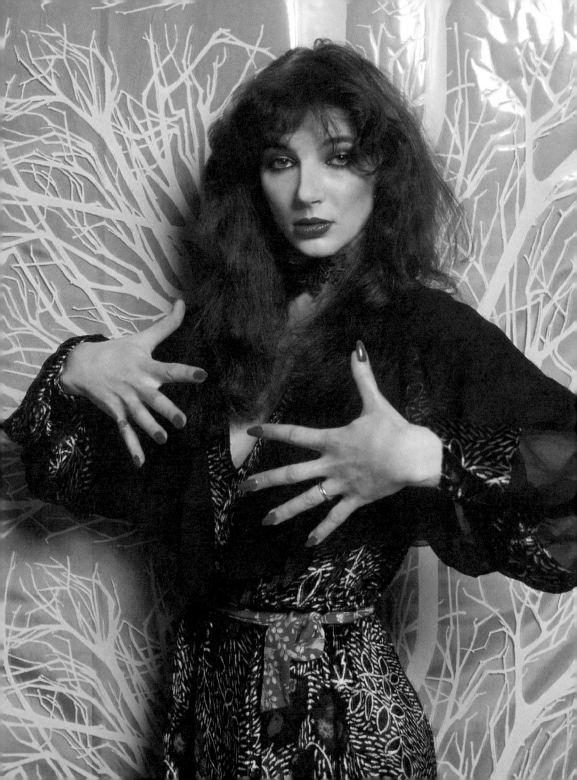

KATE BUSH

UK, born 1958

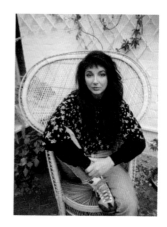

'*I just find it frustrating that people think that I'm some kind of weirdo reclusive that never comes out into the world.*'

On Thursday, 16 February 1978, Kate Bush made her television debut, singing 'Wuthering Heights' on *Top of the Pops* and looking like a modern witch. She wore an austere floor-length black figure-hugging dress, sleeves buttoned tightly at the wrists. Her halo of auburn hair was on the verge of wild, her skin pale, a single red silk rose tucked above her ear. As she crouched on the stage, the audience shuffled about looking slightly bemused. Were they supposed to dance to this?

Bush looked and sounded like a banshee, and she was singing about the hero of a gothic novel by Emily Brontë. From that point, whether hooked or completely bewildered, you were definitely haunted. Despite her contemporary dancer look and progressive sound, she became a hit machine with songs including 'The Man with the Child in his Eyes' (1978), 'Babooshka' (1980) and 'Running up that Hill' (1985).

Bush took Lycra, crystal-embellished leotards, one-shoulder catsuits and leg warmers out of the dance studio and into mainstream fashion. Occasionally there was a little crossover into the realms of disco, or a starship trooper with thigh-high boots, Russian headdresses, Japanese kimonos and fetishwear thrown in for good measure.

Writing dark songs about the female psyche and the female condition, Bush used her whole body in her performances. Only she could sing so passionately about clothes in a washing machine (metaphorically, at least), as in her song 'Mrs Bartolozzi' (2005). She was there at the beginning of the age of the pop video, and her performance-art imagery was often a little unnerving. 'Running up that Hill' is all expressionistic long shadows, contemporary dance and Japanese samurai warrior trousers. She was unashamedly sensual, art house and uncompromising. Her sex appeal was intimate and mysterious, and often she seemed to be simply off in her own sensory world, dancing through the woods in a medieval-style velvet dress with a wimple perched on her head.

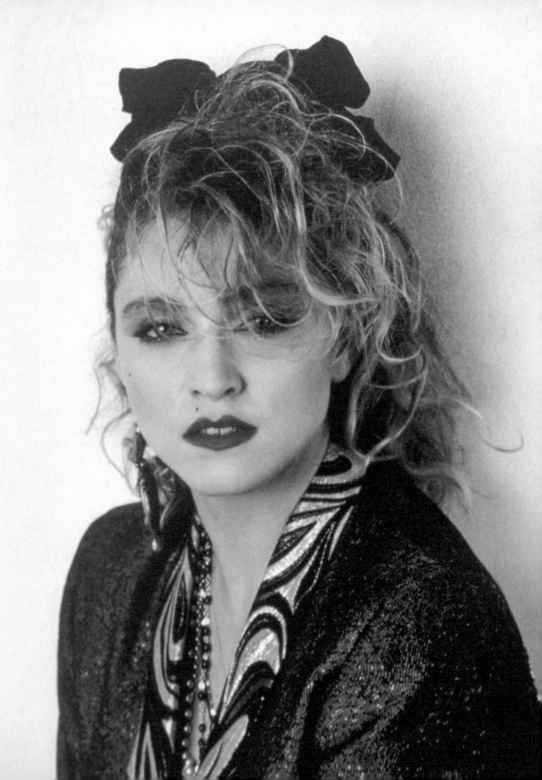

MADONNA

USA, born 1958

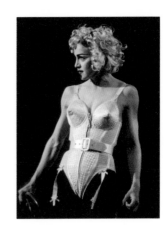

'I'm tough, I'm ambitious and I know exactly what I want. If that makes me a bitch, okay.'

When Madonna burst on to the scene in 1982 with her single 'Everybody', her unruly eyebrows, stacks of market bracelets and crucifix necklaces, and her bleached, party-girl, not-slept-for-a-week hair, she was an electrifying blast of energy. She wore ra-ra skirts over below-the-knee leggings, fishnet vests with her bra straps on show, ripped jeans over lacy tights. She had incredible charisma and was the coolest girl you could ever meet, but at the same time her look was accessible to the teenage girls around the world who had never seen anything like it. She was far from perfect, after all, and her mascara might have been a day or two old. She was sexy but streetwise, she was irreverent and oh, could she dance!

New York in the 1980s was on the edge, a near-bankrupt city with high crime, graffitied subway trains and the coolest music and art scenes mashed together in an explosion of raw, gritty creativity. Madonna arrived there in 1977, from Michigan, in search of fame and fortune, drawn to the city that had been attracting oddballs, outsiders and misfits like a magnet since the 1960s and 1970s days of punk, Studio 54 and Andy Warhol's Factory. It was a city of sexual, creative and artistic freedom, as personified by Keith Haring, Jean-Michel Basquiat and this dance-crazy, crucifix-wearing punk daughter of Roman Catholic Italian immigrants. When the song 'Like a Virgin' hit the radio shows – and, more importantly, the television screens – in 1984, Madonna's power to shock became something that she used more and more as part of her persona.

In 1985 the film *Desperately Seeking Susan* made Madonna a household name, and 'Into the Groove' became her first Number 1 hit in the UK, setting her up to become one of the bestselling pop stars of all time. Overnight, hatboxes became de rigueur as hand-bags, and Ray-Bans, headscarves and lacy tops over racy underwear influenced a generation of women (and continue to do so).

Madonna's love affair with fashion, and her ability to lead it, reached a pinnacle with the satin conical bra designed for her by Jean Paul Gaultier for the Blond Ambition World Tour in 1990. She broke many taboos about sex for women, paving the way for endless singers – from the Spice Girls to Britney Spears, Miley Cyrus and Taylor Swift – to behave as badly as they liked.

ISABELLA BLOW

UK, 1958–2007

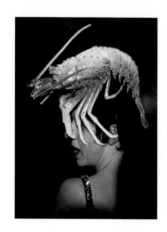

'Fashion is a vampiric thing, it's the hoover on your brain. That's why I wear the hats, to keep everyone away from me.'

One of fashion's great eccentrics, Isabella Blow was best known for her extraordinary headwear. She would wear a crystal-encrusted lobster on her head one day, a whole pheasant the next, as a way of both showing off and hiding away, making herself untouchable.

Blow started out working in New York as Anna Wintour's assistant on *Vogue* in the early 1980s, and moved to London to work with the fashion editor and photographer Michael Roberts on the *Sunday Times* and *Tatler*. She was a surrealist who was obsessed with history. Her high-drama aesthetic appealed to the designers who called her their muse, and to Lady Gaga, who regards Blow as one of her great style inspirations.

Blow's wardrobe, filled with feathers, furs, antlers, macabre references and gothic lace, was harvested from the collections of the designers she adored. She often bought clothes in instalments from student degree shows, as at the Royal College of Art in 1989, when, as style editor at *Tatler*, she adopted the milliner Philip Treacy; or at St Martins, where she discovered Alexander McQueen in 1992. She commissioned Treacy to make a headdress for her medieval-style wedding, and she became his muse as well as his greatest ambassador. She helped to promote the work of 'her' designers, creating mutually beneficial links with the more commercial side of the business, such as when she introduced McQueen to Gucci, for example.

After Blow's death in 2007, her friend Daphne Guinness bought her entire collection of clothes and accessories, including her Manolo Blahnik shoes (she would wear them mismatched); countless hats by Treacy, among them the incredible black galleon she commissioned in 1994; her collection of jewelled and sculptural sunglasses; and many rare examples of McQueen. The collection was the subject of an exhibition at Somerset House.

Blow's impact on the fashion world was that she wore these clothes that fused history and fashion in her everyday life. The avant-garde was her normal. She was a great show-woman, an ambassador for London fashion at a time when designers such as McQueen, Julien Macdonald and Hussein Chalayan were at their most experimental. She was one of the few who dared to wear some of those designers' showpieces. For Blow, though, it was not dressing up: it was her life.

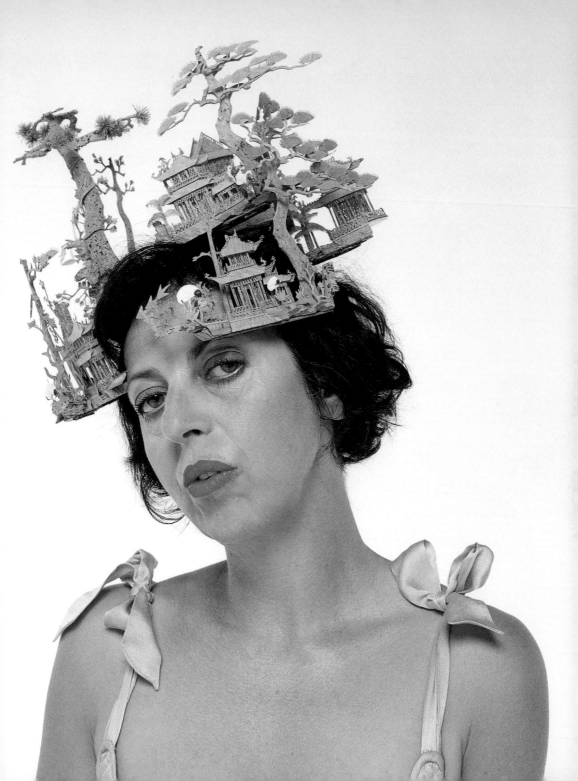

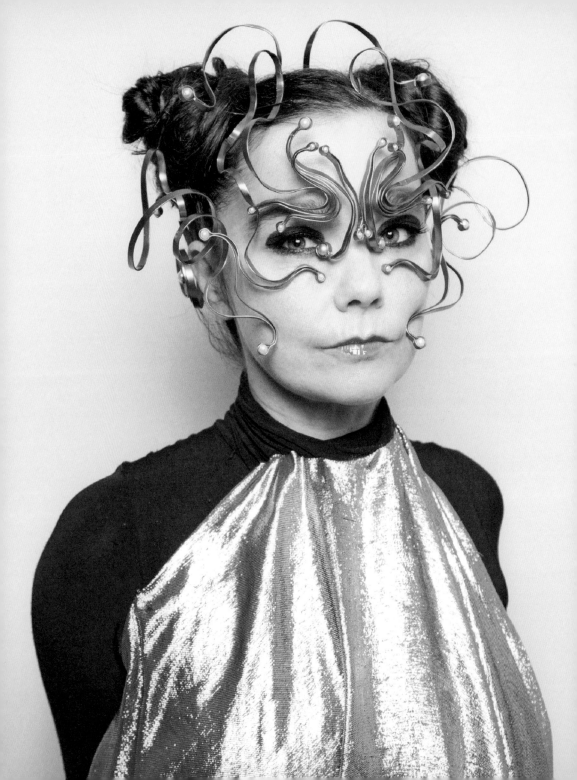

BJÖRK

Iceland, born 1965

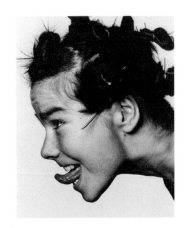

'I am one of the most idiosyncratic people around.'

Oh, Björk, where to start? The Icelandic force of nature defies all categorization; she is as much of a maverick in the way she makes music as in the way she dresses. She's as close as we can get to an alien from outer space. Everything about her is otherworldly, from the complexity of her music and vocals to her utter disregard of sartorial convention. Why not dress as a white latex orchid, complete with face mask and pearls for eyes, as she did for her Utopia Tour in 2018?

Let's run through a few of Björk's most memorable outfits. In the early days, there was a mohair jumper, its loose, hairy texture somehow accentuated by the spikes she created in her hair by rubbing in butter (or whatever grease happened to be at hand) and coiling it into knots. There was the Hussein Chalayan Airmail dress, made from unrippable envelope paper and worn (appropriately enough) for the cover of her album *Post* (1995). There was the swan dress by Marjan Pejoski, which Björk wore to the Academy Awards in 2001; the kimono dress by Alexander McQueen for the cover of *Homogenic* (2004); and the futuristic ball of quills by the milliner Maiko Takeda. Björk is as excited about new design talent as she is about new music, and her recent discoveries have included Kevin Germanier, whose final BA collection from Central Saint Martins in 2017 was made with a rainbow of recycled crystals and beads.

Björk is always ahead of the curve. She launched her website in 1994, becoming one of the first musicians to embrace the web in this way. Her album *Biophilia* (2011) came with an app for each track, and she used 360° cameras, drones and 3D printing to create an immersive experience for *Vulnicura* in 2015. The same goes for her clothes, which are always an extension of the musical experience, a mix of the new and futuristic, psychedelia, nature, folklore, ancient music, the tribal, the urban and the supernatural.

Utterly original in everything she does, Björk is never afraid of trying something new, even if there is a risk that it could be a mistake. If the results are sometimes totally bonkers, you get the impression she really couldn't care less – and that makes you love her all the more.

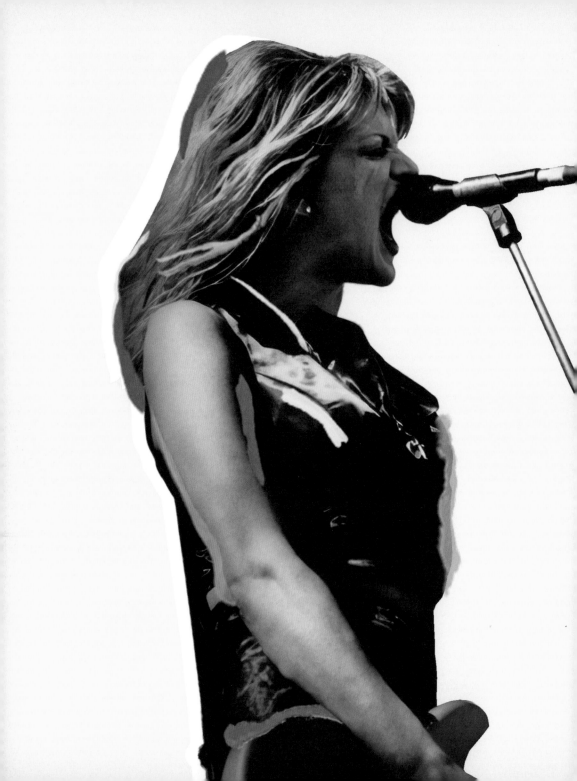

Punk Princesses

Punk is much more than a look; it's about radical thinking and a revolutionary spirit. The women in this chapter might not spike their hair or pierce their cheeks with safety pins, but they are all freethinkers, set on breaking rules and changing the status quo. And, in her own way, each of them has done that, paving the way for others to follow.

YOKO ONO

Japan, born 1933

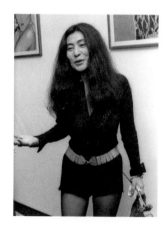

'Controversy is part of the nature of art and creativity.'

She may be a gentle punk, but Yoko Ono has always been deeply subversive: a freethinker, a misfit and anti-establishment. When she first met John Lennon in 1966, at an exhibition of her work at the Indica Gallery in London, Ono was already established as a conceptual artist in her own right. One of her most famous works is *Cut Piece*, first performed in Kyoto in 1964, in which she sits motionless and tells members of the audience to approach and cut off a piece of her clothing. They are allowed to keep the piece of cloth. The performance continues until she is almost naked and there is nothing left to cut, making it a commentary on materialism and consumerism that is still just as relevant today.

As a radical artist and activist, as well as Lennon's wife, Ono has a sense of style that has been hugely influential. She brought modernity and minimalism to fashion in the 1960s. Take her wedding outfit in 1969: a short white dress, knee-high socks and a pair of lace-up plimsolls with a wide-brimmed white hat and bug-eyed sunglasses. It's so simple, it's timeless – flower power without the flowers.

White was Ono's favourite colour, symbolic of purity, peace and power. Her exhibition at the Indica included *White Chess Set*, where all the pieces were white, turning a game of war into one of collaboration and peace. Her honeymoon with Lennon took the form of two week-long 'Bed-ins for Peace' in 1969, the first in Amsterdam protesting against the Vietnam War. The two of them dressed in white, Ono's mass of unkempt hair almost hiding her face, is a defining image of the period.

Ono was – and still is – the personification of the avant-garde and an activist for social change and feminism. Despite being wheelchair-bound, she attended the Women's March in 2017 holding a placard with the words 'Imagine Peace', combining her two main areas of activism: feminism and world peace.

With her make-up-free face (she doesn't even like the feel of moisturizer) and oversized visor sunglasses, Ono never seems to age. Hats are a signature of her look, whether a bowler hat, top hat or beret, and a reminder of her ongoing nonconformism.

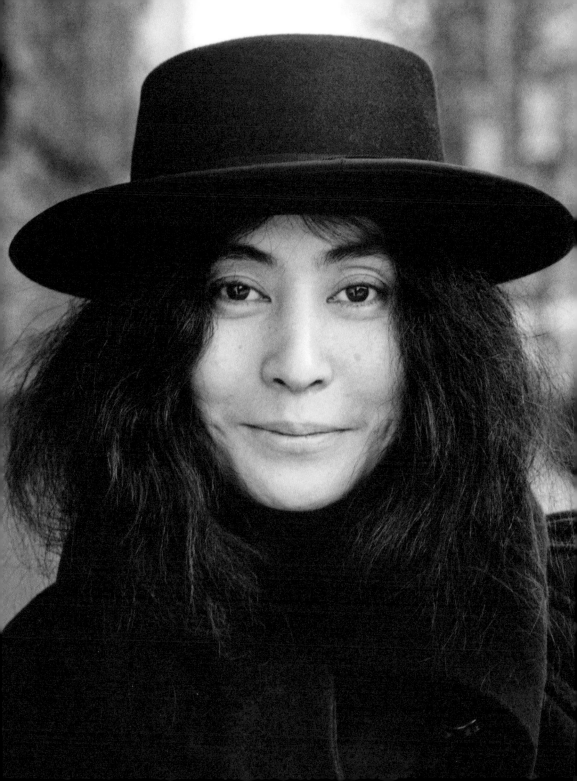

VIVIENNE
WESTWOOD

UK, born 1941

'I'm a punk because I'm a fighter. I can't help it.'

She's the woman who dressed the punk rock movement. She opened her first shop, Let It Rock, with her then boyfriend Malcolm McLaren in London in 1971, and the world has not been the same since. They started out selling clothes inspired by 1950s rock 'n' roll. In 1973 the shop became Too Fast to Live, Too Young to Die, selling clothes as a weapon for being sexually aggressive and politically provocative, a massive two fingers to anyone in power, from politicians and royalty to the British class system. The following year the shop changed its name to Sex, with a focus on rubber and fetishwear, and in 1976 it became Seditionaries, offering the full-on punk look. This was the style – and social scene – that gave birth to the Sex Pistols. Rips, studs, safety pins, pornographic imagery and bondage were all Westwood and McLaren's inventions.

In the 1980s Westwood's collections spearheaded the New Romantic movement; her first proper fashion collection was 'Pirates' (Autumn/Winter 1981), a mix of tricorn highwayman hats and military uniforms, featuring a squiggly print smocked shirt. The look was made popular by bands such as Adam and the Ants and Bow Wow Wow. Her collections during that decade included 'Nostalgia of Mud' (sometimes called 'Buffalo Girls') in 1982 (Pharrell Williams revived the Buffalo hat when he wore it in 2014), 'Witches' the following year, with prints by Keith Haring, and the famous puffball mini-crini of 1985, which became the silhouette of the late 1980s, borrowed by Christian Lacroix and copied endlessly on the high street. Westwood gave us the elevator shoe, the rocking-horse shoe and stilettos with studs, reinterpreted the twinset and subverted the cocktail dress to make it the wrong side of sexy, designed to be worn – as she prefers – without undergarments. Her corsets, inspired by eighteenth-century underwear, have become a wardrobe staple.

It is impossible to underestimate the influence Westwood has had on our wardrobes, as well as on the way we think about fashion. Since 2015 she has been a member of the Green Party in the UK, and she actively campaigns against nuclear weapons and for the combating of climate change. She continues to use the subversive power of fashion, leading the way for a new generation of activists.

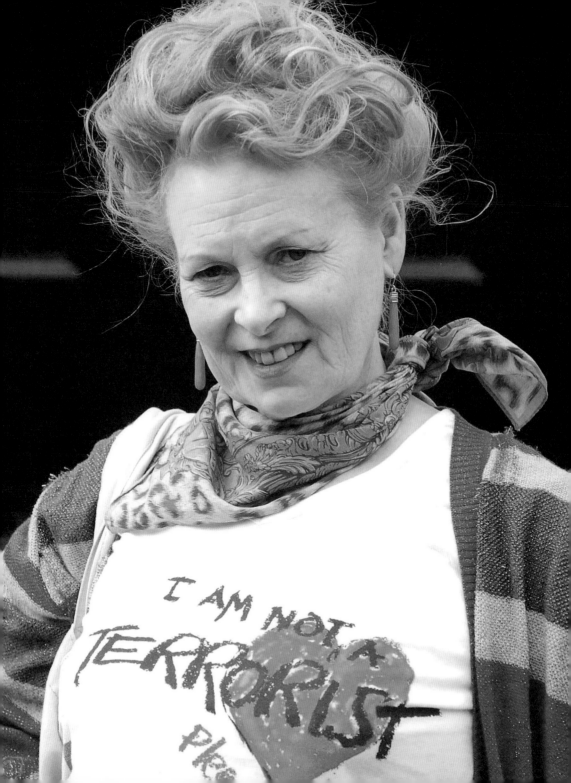

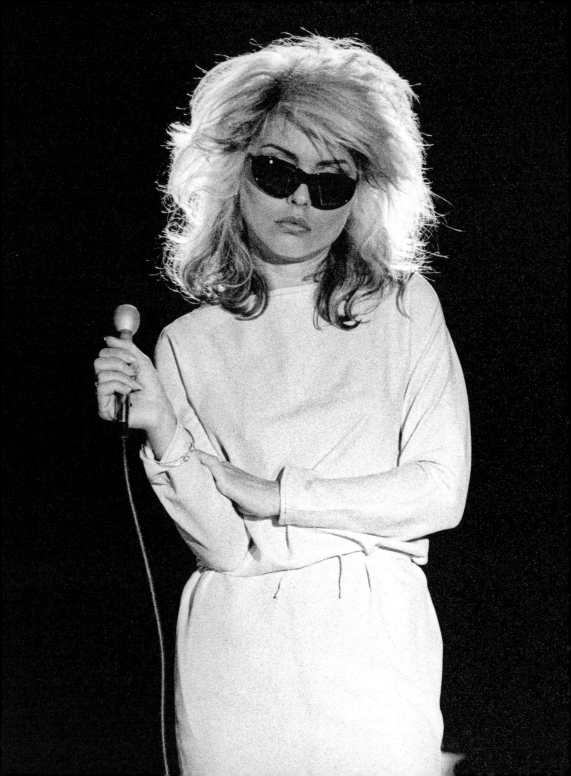

DEBBIE HARRY

USA, born 1945

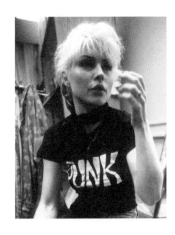

'The only person I really believe in is me.'

With the highest cheekbones in the business, and the shortest skirts, Debbie Harry mixed sex kitten with spiky punk. She could veer from airbrushed glamour – glossy lips, blue eyeshadow and one-shoulder dresses – to dominatrix in thigh-high red boots.

Harry formed the band Blondie in 1974 with Chris Stein, who had joined Harry's first band, the Stilettos, in 1973. Harry and her bandmates were regulars at the legendary New York club CBGB, and were friends with bands like the Ramones and Lou Reed's Velvet Underground, and with David Bowie. They were pure downtown New York punk glamour.

There was little difference between Harry's Andy Warhol screen print and the real thing. She would wear her own homemade fashion creations: a boob tube that looked as though it had been sewn with shards of glass, worn in the video for 'Rapture' (1980), in which she experimented with early rap; a dress made from double-sided razor blades that she said looked like snakeskin; an orange boiler suit and aviator sunglasses. She had a cool line in T-shirts, too. For an appearance on *Top of the Pops* in the UK in February 1978, singing 'Denis', she wore nothing but an oversized shirt and a pair of thigh-high boots.

Harry's hair was bleached blonde with darker streaks underneath, and you were never sure if she'd just bleached it badly like the punk she was. In some ways she was a warped version of Marilyn Monroe (see page 112), the darker, younger sister who had been led astray. She had candyfloss hair and the most seductive of pouts, even when she appeared to be wearing a black bin bag (at her most sexily subversive in the video for 'Atomic', 1979, over a ripped T-shirt tucked into a pair of tights). But she was always powerful. 'I felt women should not portray themselves as victims. We were counterculture of the period,' she told the BBC's *Desert Island Discs* in 2011 in a programme that is really worth a listen.

Harry paved the way for endless nonconformists after her, from Madonna (see page 51) to Courtney Love (see page 73), the fashion designer Pam Hogg and Beth Ditto (see page 75).

MARIANNE FAITHFULL

UK, born 1946

'Rebellion is the only thing that keeps you alive!'

She's not a punk in the conventional sense of the word, but Marianne Faithfull has an underlying punk spirit, a devil-may-care attitude that has both got her into trouble and made her one of life's most inspiring survivors. She was the figurehead of the counterculture in 1960s London, a time when youth, hedonism, bohemia and freedom were everything. She had 'The Look' of the decade: the blond hair, the big, daydreamy eyes, the soft, pouty mouth and a style all her own. She could sing, too. She had been training to be an opera singer, but fell instead into the world of rock 'n' roll – well, more folk 'n' roll – with the single 'As Tears Go By' (1964) and her first album, *Come My Way*, released in 1965.

Faithfull's relationship with Mick Jagger began in 1966 – the year after she had married artist John Dunbar, the father of her child – and was followed by an infamous drugs bust at Keith Richards's estate in Sussex and a role as the leather-clad star of *Girl on a Motorcycle* (or *Naked Under Leather*; 1968), all of which sealed her reputation as the most infamous rock chick in the history of infamous rock chicks. Faithfull played the role perfectly, her long, fringed hair and her clothes tinged with the hippy trail. It's still a look that women love to copy – essentially the uniform of Coachella – worn by everyone from her friend Kate Moss to Gigi Hadid (see pages 22 and 28).

After she left Jagger in 1970, and lost custody of her son, Faithfull's life took a downward turn, resulting in drug addiction, attempted suicide and homelessness in the 1970s. But in 1979, the year she married Ben Brierley of the punk band the Vibrators, she made a comeback with the hit song 'Broken English', the sweetness of her voice roughened by the life she had led. She hadn't got stuck in a 1960s time warp: when she performed on television, she did so dressed in an industrial post-punk pink boiler suit, like Debbie Harry's older, world-weary big sister (see previous page), but totally of her time. It's a dark, haunting song, inspired by the German terrorist gang the Baader-Meinhof Group.

Faithfull now lives in Ireland, still writing and still recording, playing music loud in the early hours, and doing just what she likes.

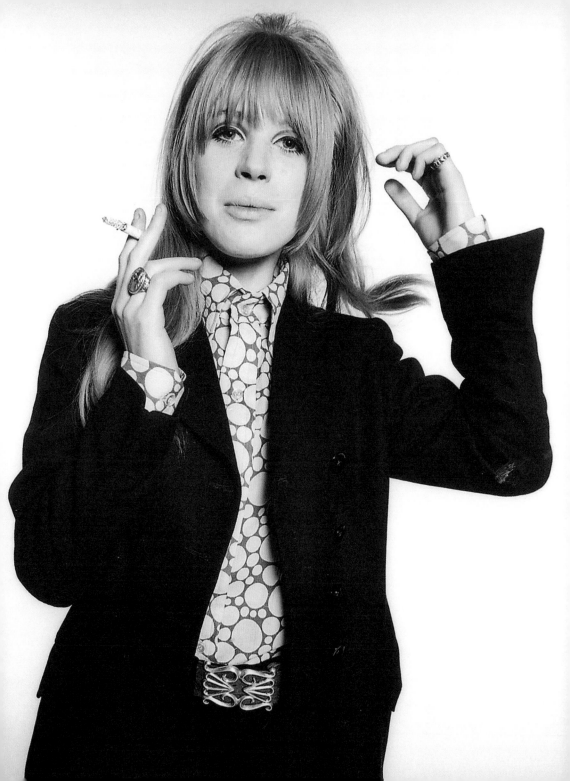

PATTI SMITH

USA, born 1946

'My style says, "Look at me, don't look at me."'

P atti Smith has never been actively interested in fashion, but somehow fashion keeps catching up with her, falling in love with her androgyny, the way she would tie a black ribbon round the collar of her shirt or sling her jacket over her shoulder Frank Sinatra-style. It's a state of mind more than a sense of fashion. The photograph on the cover of her 1975 album *Horses*, taken by her then boyfriend, Robert Mapplethorpe, changed the course of fashion. The white shirt she wore in the picture was – like most of Smith's clothes at the time – from the Salvation Army in the Bowery. It was, she said, just the way she dressed.

As well as signalling the beginning of punk music, then, that album gave women a new, androgynous way of dressing. For Smith, dungarees, pegged trousers, men's shirts and jackets were just what she felt comfortable in; they were her work clothes. The fashion designer Hedi Slimane photographed Kate Moss (see page 22) and Jamie Bochert in homage to the singer for *Vogue* in 2010. You feel her spirit in his work for Saint Laurent, and it will no doubt feature for Céline after he became the label's creative director in 2018. Phoebe Philo (see page 92) is another fan, as is Paul Smith, who

devoted a collection to Smith. Margaret Howell counts Smith in her top three style icons, and Smith's independent spirit, simplicity and androgyny recur in the designer's tomboyish collections.

As a teenager, the Belgian designer Ann Demeulemeester was entranced by the *Horses* image. When she began designing her own collections in 1985, she sent Smith three white shirts she had made, and the two women became friends. 'Freedom exists in the soul of one's work,' Smith later said of Demeulemeester. 'Ann bequeaths this intangible aspect to the wearer.' As one of the most influential designers of the 1990s, Demeulemeester reworked Smith's linear look over and over again, making it a uniform for the fashionable intellectuals of the decade.

Smith's hair – centre-parted, choppy, unkempt – has had a huge influence, too. There's a powerful picture of her in 1978 staring into the camera lens, about to cut her own hair. The resulting jagged haircut, the unruly brows, the stark gaze were all about attitude – either you have it or you don't. Of course, Smith had it in buckets. Her style seemed to come not from the clothes themselves but from somewhere deeper within.

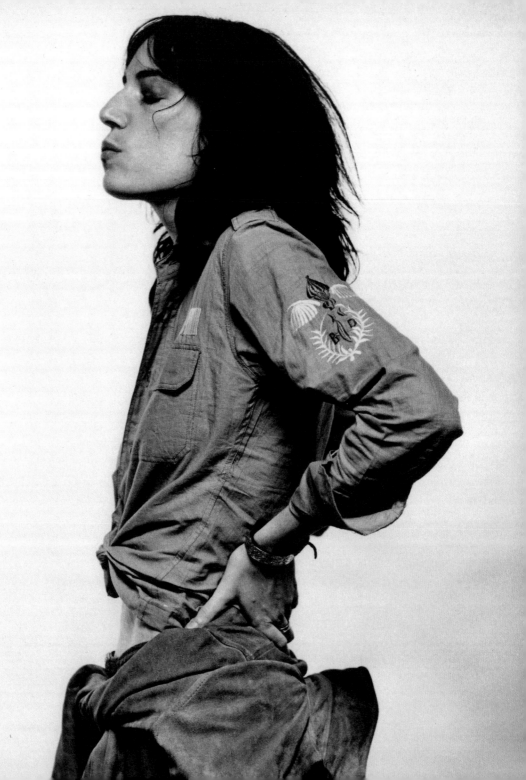

POLY STYRENE

UK, 1957–2011

*'I said that I wasn't a sex symbol
and that if anybody tried to make
me one I'd shave my head tomorrow.'*

With metal braces cemented to her teeth, jangly, brightly coloured earrings and an apparent indifference to conventional sex appeal, Poly Styrene was the most unlikely of pop stars. She was a unique talent who has inspired generations of women not to cave in to convention.

At the age of 19, Styrene (born Marianne Joan Elliott-Said) advertised in *Melody Maker* and *NME* for 'Young Punx who want to stick it together'. The result was the new-wave band X-Ray Spex, named after Styrene's American GI aunt sent her a pair of novelty X-Ray glasses in the post. Her own name came from a flick through the Yellow Pages. 'I chose the name Poly Styrene because it's a lightweight, disposable product,' she said, 'a send-up of a pop star, just plastic, disposable.'

Much of what Styrene did was about sending things up, including herself in her song 'I am a Cliché' (1978). She had a wry sense of humour and a sharp eye for everyday life going on around her. The band's debut single, 'Oh Bondage Up Yours' (1977), was written after seeing two girls chained together at a gig. It was, Styrene said later, about slavery and the suffragettes

as well as the clothes in the window of Vivienne Westwood's shop Seditionaries (see page 60).

Reporters at the time liked to infer that Styrene's references to brightly coloured plastic were a code for LSD, but in fact she simply had a genuine fascination with kitsch plastic and Day-Glo clothes. For a while, she had a stall at Beaufort Market in Chelsea, the epicentre of punk London in the mid-1970s, selling trashy plastic accessories, army surplus and brightly coloured clothes. Her style included smart army-surplus jackets with lots of gold frogging, oddball helmets and the odd 1960s skirt suit. Nothing was bought new.

Styrene, who tuned into mindless consumerism long before it was mainstream, was far ahead of her time. Her lyrics about supermarkets, plastic, Kleenex and Weetabix ('Plastic Bag', 1977) – and obsessive cleanliness and SR toothpaste in her best-known song, 'Germ Free Adolescents' – were brilliantly observed, their details far more subtle, domestic and subversively feminist than anything that is usually associated with punk rock.

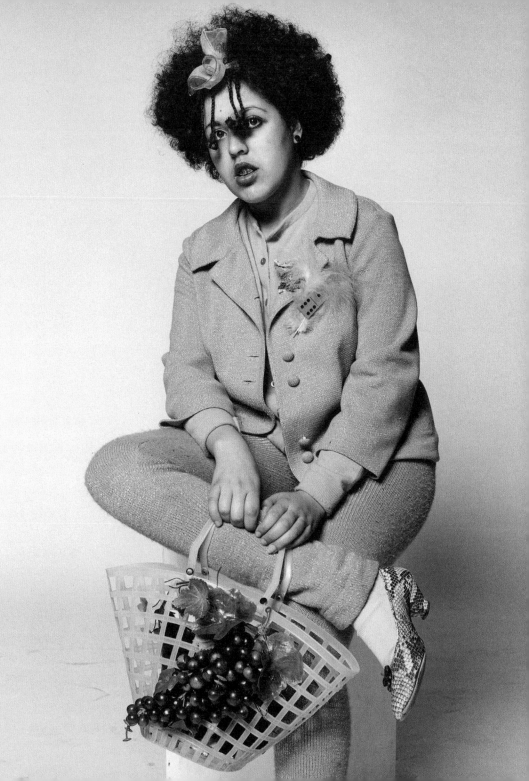

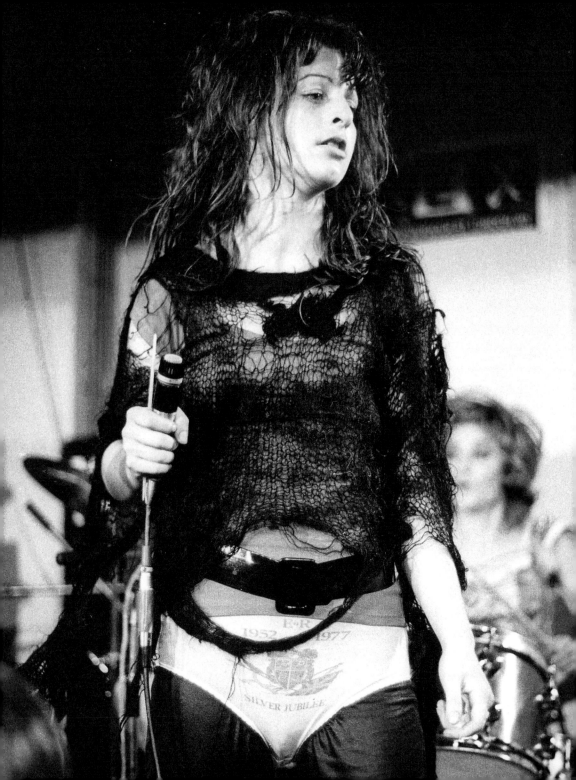

ARI UP

Germany, 1962–2010

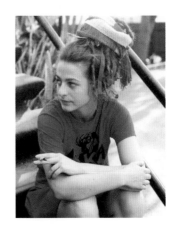

'Find out who you really are, then accept who you are. Fight for your life every day to be who you are.'

A ri Up was the ultimate teenage rebel. Her unfettered performances as singer of the all-girl punk band the Slits would have been unsettling for a grown woman, but she formed the band at the height of punk rock in 1976, when she was just 14. When the Slits supported the Clash on their White Riot Tour of 1977, her underage status simply added to the shock of seeing a group of girls on stage, seemingly not in control of themselves, their ripped-up school uniforms or their instruments. Where was her mother, you might well ask? Well, Nora Forster was a music promoter, regularly entertaining rock stars, such as members of The Clash, at home. It was she who introduced the impressionable Ari (born Ariane Daniela Forster) to the world of punk rock when she took her to see the Sex Pistols play in 1975 (Nora went on to marry Johnny Rotten).

The Slits' album *Cut* (1979), produced by Dennis Bovell, was a mix of punk and reggae and has since become seminal. Ari Up's impact was to make it fine to be a teenage dirtbag (at least, fine to all the other delinquent teenagers who were watching and waiting for a sign), to make it quite all right to stand up on stage without being able to sing – even remotely – in tune (if the boys could do it, why couldn't the girls?). She made it OK to be a female punk rocker in a male-dominated world, to behave as badly as the boys, to make up her own rules about just about everything – and then to break them like a true anarchist.

Ari Up did all this in shredded mohair jumpers, crude make-up, ragged clothes and shrunken school blazers, with matted hair. She was the DIY queen before customization was even a thing. She wore her knickers over her tights and danced as though she was possessed. She was rude and crude, and she really didn't care what anyone thought. For that, we will be forever grateful.

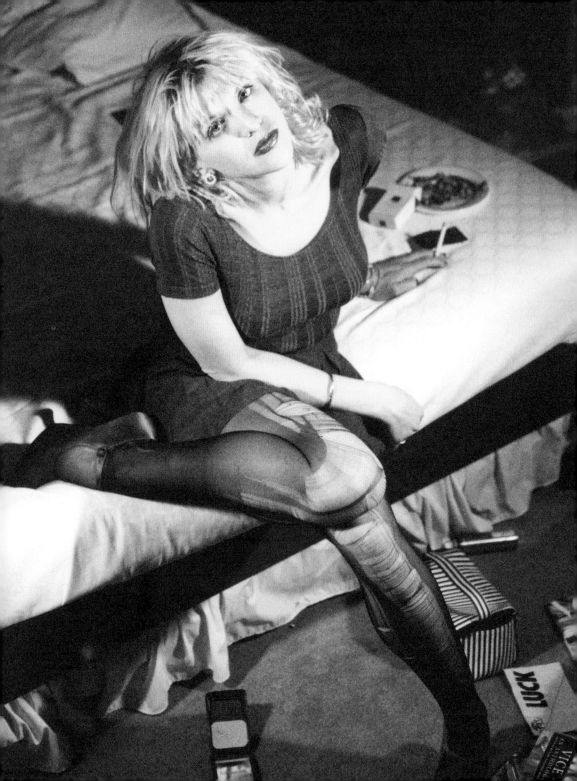

COURTNEY LOVE

USA, born 1964

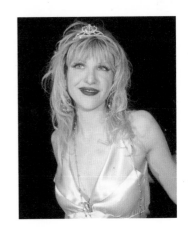

'From David Bowie, I knew you had to have a look and a hair style ... so I kind of invented one.'

Baby-doll dresses, Peter Pan collars, miniature tiaras and trashy make-up spell only one thing: Courtney Love. For much of the early 1990s, Love had the Look. All you needed was a silky slip dress, heavily laddered tights, enough mascara to look as though you had been crying half the night, red lips – and pale Pan-Cake to cover your zits. Blonde hair, a tiny tiara or your little sister's plastic hairslide and the words 'witch' or 'slut' scrawled on your arms were optional.

In 1989 Love advertised for band members ('I want to start a band. My influences are Big Black, Stooges, Sonic Youth and Fleetwood Mac') and started to perform as part of Hole, in grimy vintage dresses, as though she were a prom princess who had gone off the rails. Hole's debut album, *Pretty on the Inside* (1991), perfectly represented the group's warts-and-all approach to music – and to life in general. It was hard to listen to, just as Love's car-crash life and heroin addiction were hard to watch. In the man's world of rock, she showed that women could behave just as badly (if not worse), play just as violently (if not louder and more aggressively), and inspire million-dollar bidding wars between record labels. When she signed with the same label as Nirvana, she insisted on more money and better publishing rights. The phrase 'gender pay gap' was not in her vocabulary.

As the poster girl for grunge, Love was the inspiration for Marc Jacobs's Spring/Summer 1993 collection for Perry Ellis, complete with holey jumpers, tartan shirts, knitted beanie hats, droopy tea dresses and Dr. Martens boots. She and her husband, Kurt Cobain, were like royalty. Their fans worshipped everything about them, from their sex, drugs and rock 'n' roll lifestyles to their baby, Frances Bean. The couple carried her around with them as though she were a miniature roadie. They lived their lives publicly; no misdemeanour was hidden.

Love continues to inspire. In 2013 Hedi Slimane photographed her in gritty black and white for an advertising campaign for Saint Laurent. In a world that is full of plastic, Courtney Love is about as real as it gets.

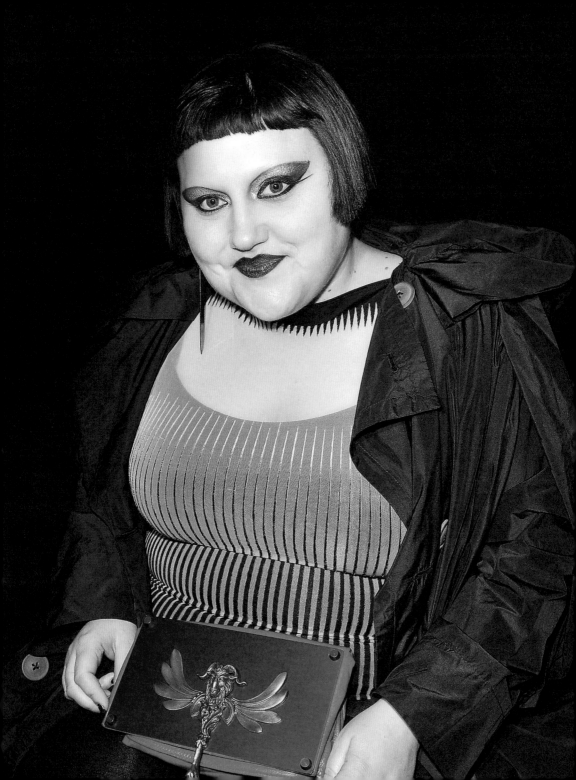

BETH
DITTO

USA, born 1981

'*I have no control over what people
think of me but I have 100% control
over what I think of myself.*'

Among many things, Beth Ditto considers herself a punk. Not in the Mohicanned, safety-pinned-cheek kind of way, but within her own subgenre where punks are fat (her preferred adjective, in her opinion far preferable to the polite 'curvy'), outspoken, lesbian, nonconformist, feminist and, if they like, wear frocks made by Karl Lagerfeld or Jean Paul Gaultier, who made her wedding dress. She doesn't shave her armpits or wear deodorant because she says punks should smell.

Ditto's fatness has certainly been a talking point. In 2009 she told *BlackBook*: 'It's kind of like a drug … it's a performance. It's funny how something so normal and mundane that you see every day – your body – can be controversial. The shock value is intense. It's like carrying an art piece around with you all the time.' She has her own quaintly old-school notions of classic all-out glamour-girl beauty – she never does anything without eyeliner and lipstick – has modelled for *Dazed*, *Love* (naked) and *Vogue*, and walked down the catwalk for Marc Jacobs and Jean Paul Gaultier and for Alexander Wang's Do Something campaign.

Ditto's style inspirations are many – Siouxsie Sioux, Greta Garbo, Poly Styrene, Cyndi Lauper (see pages 174, 105, 70 and 209), Boy George – but her light-bulb moment came when she discovered the punk feminist Riot Grrrl movement, which legitimized her desire to wear lipstick, a baby-doll dress and Converse, and ride a skateboard. She didn't have to shave her legs if she wore a dress, but she could still wear a girly hairslide. Beauty and femininity mean many different things, but she believes being interesting is what really counts.

In 2009 Ditto launched her eponymous collection for the British high-street chain Evans, aimed at women with as much confidence as her, who also happen to be a size 14–32. Her own collection followed in 2016, with print motifs taken from the world of cosmetics. For Ditto, dressing is about celebrating and accentuating what you've got.

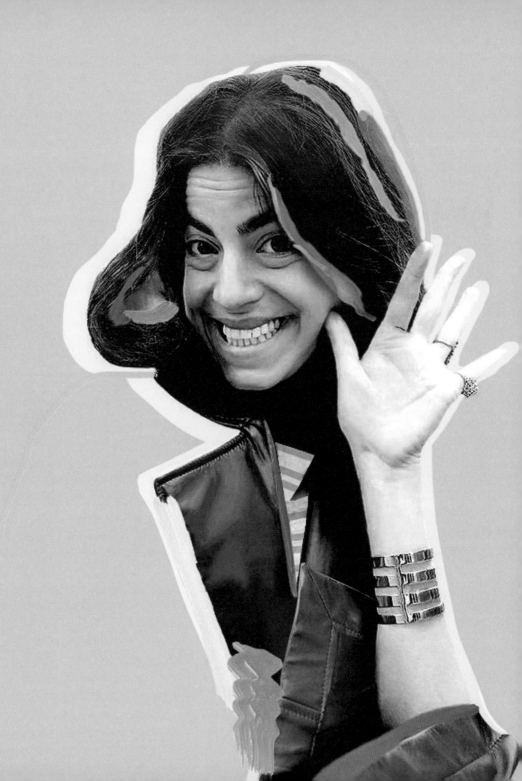

Fashion Girlfriends

Fashion girlfriends are the inspirational designers, stylists and entrepreneurs who take you on the journey with them, sharing their style and vision. These women are full of honest advice, and feel approachable enough to turn to when you don't know what to wear or how to wear it. Fashion girlfriends are there to fill you with confidence and make you feel better about yourself – whether through an encouraging comment on Instagram or passing on a tip from their own experience. They know what they're talking about, so look and learn.

COCO CHANEL

France, 1883–1971

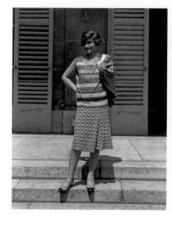

'It is always better to be slightly underdressed.'

I t has to be said that Gabrielle 'Coco' Chanel was more at home in the company of men, but she did have a close friendship (possibly a love affair) with Misia Sert, the well-connected, opium-addicted pianist, patron of the arts and celebrated artists' muse. They met at a dinner party in 1917, and Chanel is believed to have designed the pink dress that Sert was buried in in 1950.

On the whole, though, Chanel was not your typical BFF; in fact, most sensible women would probably run a mile from her caustic wit. What endeared her to the women whose wardrobes she helped to revolutionize was the liberation from the early twentieth-century constraints of the corset and starchy petticoats, the shortening of skirts to make them easier to move in, the suntan – she made a bronzed Riviera complexion fashionable – and the introduction of practical knitwear. Chanel made it fashionable to dress in a more pared-down way, and led by example, wearing trousers, sailor's tops, jerseys and blazers. For her, it was all about simplicity: form always had to follow function, and she insisted that luxury could be comfortable.

Perhaps surprisingly, Chanel was not born into privileged social circles. Her mother died when she was 12, and she was subsequently raised in an orphanage run by nuns. It was there that she learned to sew, but it was a strict, austere life. Her big break came when she met Captain Arthur Edward 'Boy' Capel, who was the love of her life until his untimely death in a car accident in 1919. He financed Chanel's business, allowing her to open shops in Paris, Deauville and Biarritz between 1910 and 1915.

Chanel's success continued with the introduction of the fragrance Chanel No. 5 in 1921. She also gave us many of the classics we rely on today: the universal little black dress in 1926, designed to fit and flatter all women; traditional British fabrics such as tweed for skirt suits, the jacket tailored softly as a cardigan, and weighted down by a chain around the hem to make it hang just perfectly; and costume jewellery, which she loved and wore as though it were made of precious pearls and diamonds. In 1955 Chanel gave us the quilted 2.55 handbag with its distinctive gold chain – a timeless classic whose tangible glamour will never fade.

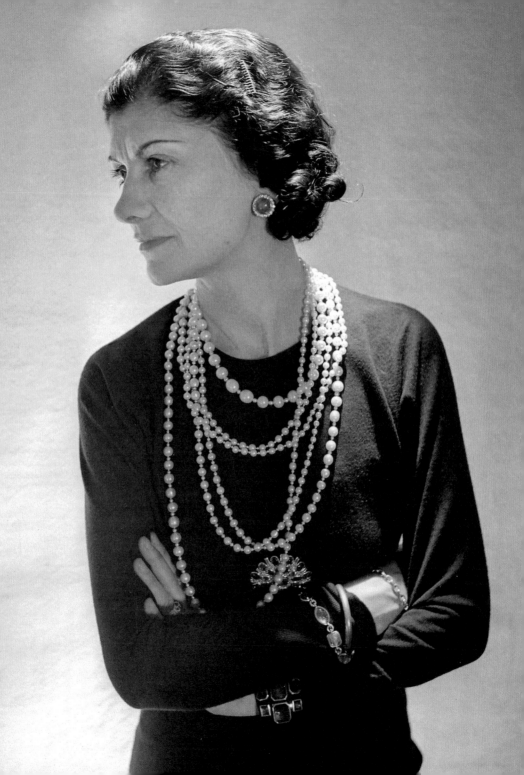

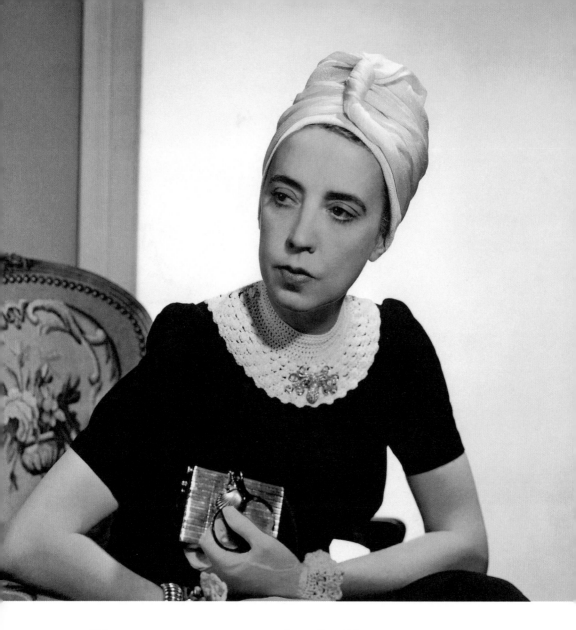

'Ninety per cent are afraid of being conspicuous,
and of what people say. So they buy a grey suit.
They should dare to be different.'

ELSA SCHIAPARELLI

Italy, 1890–1973

E lsa Schiaparelli was the best fashion girlfriend you could hope for. She was full of smart advice on how to dress, and she even came up with 12 Commandments to help you on your way (Number 5 is quoted opposite).

Schiaparelli lived through one of the most extraordinary periods of modern history, and made a mark so indelible and so vibrant that she remains one of fashion's most enduring influences. She tapped into the mood of the times, whether it was whimsical knitwear (her famous Bow Knot sweater, with its playful *trompe l'œil* sailor collar and bow, became a popular knitting pattern in America) or the revolutionary zip, which eliminated the need for fiddly hooks and eyes and buttons. She understood the power of the accessory, especially if it were a bag shaped like a lobster, a shoe worn as a hat, large buttons shaped as vanity mirrors, or a perfume bottle in the shape of Mae West's nude torso. Her foreboding Tear Dress (1938) with its *trompe l'œil* 'torn' fabric has been seen as positively punk.

Although she dressed a great many influential women of her time – from Marlene Dietrich (see page 102) to Wallis Simpson (see page 184), for whose trousseau she designed 18 outfits, including the symbolic Lobster dress – Schiaparelli was her own best advertisement. Described as *jolie laide* (pretty-ugly), she was perhaps the original Man Repeller. You needed a certain playful personality to pull off some of her designs, and only she could get away with dressing up as an eighteenth-century Venetian pageboy for a themed ball.

Schiaparelli introduced art to fashion, from the sophisticated painterly palette of colours she used – including her most famous, shocking pink – to the dream-like ideas she shared with the surrealist art movement of the time. The artists Salvador Dalí and Alberto Giacometti, the photographer Man Ray and the playwright Jean Cocteau were her friends and collaborators.

Schiaparelli used fashion both as a form of fantastic escapism – with collections themed on the circus or the zodiac – and to improve women's lives by making them look individual, confident and elegant. She believed not in forcing their bodies to fit into a dress, but in allowing the dress to frame the body. She closed her house in 1954, but continued (and continues) to be an inspiration to generations of designers, from Yves Saint Laurent to Jean Paul Gaultier, Martin Margiela, Miuccia Prada (see page 91) and Alexander McQueen.

CLAIRE McCARDELL

USA, 1905–1958

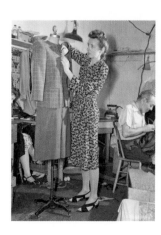

C laire McCardell was the wise, cool, brilliant big sister of fashion. Few American designers of the twentieth and twenty-first centuries will not lay down their allegiance to this most revolutionary designer, a visionary who knew that by responding to her own needs she was providing solutions for millions of other women.

McCardell created contemporary fashion, the idea of American sportswear, or clothes for everyday living. She invented the wardrobe for the modern woman who worked, played sport, cooked dinner for friends at home and took her kids to the beach at the weekend. Her tent-like Monastic Dress of 1938 did away with the constrictions of darts and waistlines, using the bias-cut grain of the fabric instead to create drape and shape.

In 1942 McCardell did it again, creating the timeless and classic Popover Dress. A wrap-around denim dress (three decades ahead of Diane von Furstenberg; see page 197), it was easy to wash and wear, and was designed to be worn over smarter clothes, targeting women who no longer had help at home because their domestic helpers were all required for wartime factory work. The designer understood perfectly how to mix utility and femininity to make clothes that answered a practical need rather than a fantasy.

McCardell developed her craft at the School of Fine and Applied Art (now Parsons) in New York. There, she bought Paris couture hand-me-downs from wealthier students, took them apart and studied them. She spent her second year in Paris, where she was influenced by Madeleine Vionnet and realized the importance not just of how clothes worked but of how they felt to wear.

In the 1930s and 1940s American fashions were dictated by those coming from Paris. For a while McCardell worked for the fashion entrepreneur Hattie Carnegie, who sent her to Paris to copy what she saw there, but McCardell simplified the designs and transformed them into clothes made from fabrics stolen from menswear and workwear, such as cotton shirting and denim. She added details such as hooks and eyes, and double rows of topstitching borrowed from Levi's jeans. Thanks to her, American designers had an entirely new vocabulary, including hooded jumpers (the precursor to today's ubiquitous hoodie – thank you, Claire); the ballet pump (often in a fabric that matched the dress, as a response to the rationing of leather during the war); and the shirt dress, still a wardrobe staple today. These were clothes that were affordable and accessible – and which also happened to transform the lives of millions of women.

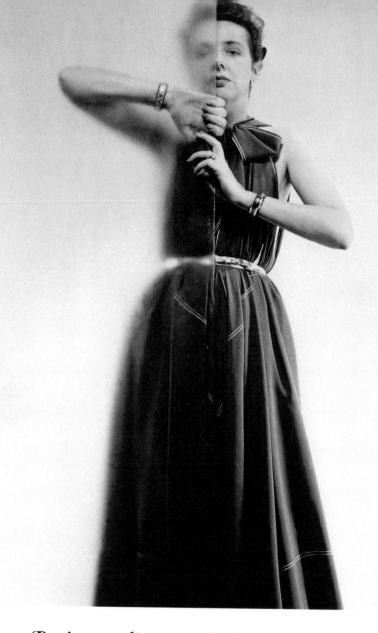

'Don't try to live up to Fashion. First of all, stay firmly you. And if Fashion seems to be saying something that isn't right for you, ignore it.'

MARY QUANT

UK, born 1934

'The point of clothes for women should be:
1) you are noticed;
2) you look sexy;
3) you feel good.'

It is almost impossible to imagine the fuss caused by Mary Quant's pioneering miniskirt. (Let's say she was the originator of the miniskirt; she certainly coined the name after her favourite car, the Mini Cooper, which appeared in 1961.) The images of her and her fellow Chelsea Girls look so innocent, with their short skirts, knee-high socks or boots and upbeat smiles. But Quant's invention had a seismic effect on society, an emblem of the revolutionary Youthquake. 'The young will not be dictated to … They will not accept truisms or propaganda,' she wrote in her autobiography *Quant by Quant* (1965).

One of the earliest fault lines of the Youthquake was Bazaar on Kings Road, Chelsea. This was the boutique started in 1955 by Mary Quant and her husband, Alexander Plunkett-Green, who also ran a restaurant, Alexander's, in the basement. During the day the shop was buzzing with young women eager to buy one of Quant's fresh, new, simple designs, many of which fastened with a daringly placed zip that could open to the navel. In the evening Alexander's was a hotspot for all the cool photographers, models and pop stars to gather to see and be seen. For a post-war society coming out of rationing and still rooted in old-fashioned formality and strict class structure, Quant was as subversive and disruptive as Vivienne Westwood (see page 60) would be with punk in the 1970s.

Quant said she created the miniskirt so that women could go about their lives with as much freedom as they needed. It was a form of liberation, both sexually and politically. Compared to the padded, corseted looks of the 1947 New Look and the stiff constriction of much of 1950s fashion, the miniskirt seemed simple and fresh and could be worn with the new tights that Quant also designed (she later diversified into make-up, footwear and even homewares). It was a world away from the grand couture of traditional high society. Quant's clothes had a sense of humour and a shoulder-shrugging, bob-flicking flippancy that reflected her personality.

The miniskirt democratized fashion. These were clothes you could try on in the shop and buy off the peg, for not too much money. A planned show at the Victoria and Albert Museum in London in 2019 and a call-out to the public to share their Quant wardrobe treasures has revived interest in Quant, and is proof that she paved the way for fashion to be for the many, not just the privileged few.

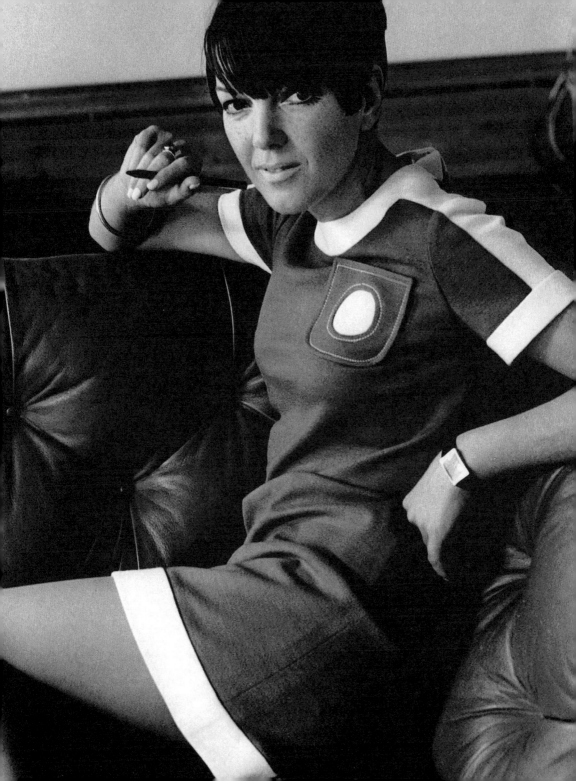

GRACE CODDINGTON

UK, born 1941

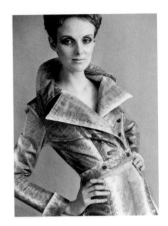

'I still weave dreams, finding inspiration wherever I can and looking for romance in the real, not the digital, world.'

Grace Coddington is a creative chameleon who can swap her style from romantic 1920s boudoir one day to contemporary cool the next. For almost 30 years she ruled over the *Vogue* fashion cupboard, scouring the designers' rails each season for the looks that would both inspire readers and spark her own vivid imagination. In the days of unlimited expense accounts, she would take her chosen photographer and their team off for weeks on end to far-flung corners of the world in search of the right location to create the perfect picture. The way she saw a season became the way the rest of the world saw it.

Coddington's own style, however, is very predictable, rather like a uniform. Her shirts are made for her by Prada, on repeat order. 'They tend to be black or white,' she said in 2015, 'but occasionally I have shirts in very bright colours. It's not very interesting the way I dress these days. I'm too old and I look stupid if I do something too clever.' Back in the 1980s her uniform was Calvin Klein, Azzedine Alaïa and Prada. More recently she has moved on to Phoebe Philo's Céline (see page 92), always in black or navy blue, with clean, unfussy lines.

Coddington prefers to remain behind the camera. But with her flame-orange hair and her famous cats (Bart and Pumpkin), she emerged as the star of the documentary *The September Issue* (2009), where she appeared strangely unfazed by the madness of the fashion industry around her.

Coddington's career has spanned six decades: beginning as a model in the late 1950s, she was then junior fashion editor of British *Vogue* and creative director of American *Vogue* twenty years later. Working with photographers including Norman Parkinson, Guy Bourdin, Helmut Newton, Steven Meisel and Bruce Weber, she has produced many of the most memorable fashion images of the twentieth and twenty-first centuries, drawing on her mix of romance and realism.

What makes Coddington such a great stylist is her innate understanding of fashion, from her early days poring over copies of *Vogue* as a teenager in Anglesey, Wales, to her time as a model in 1960s London (she was the original model for Vidal Sassoon's radical five-point bob), to knowing how to do her own make-up and style herself. She has lived life on the front line of fashion for so long that fashion is not even second nature: it's simply who she is.

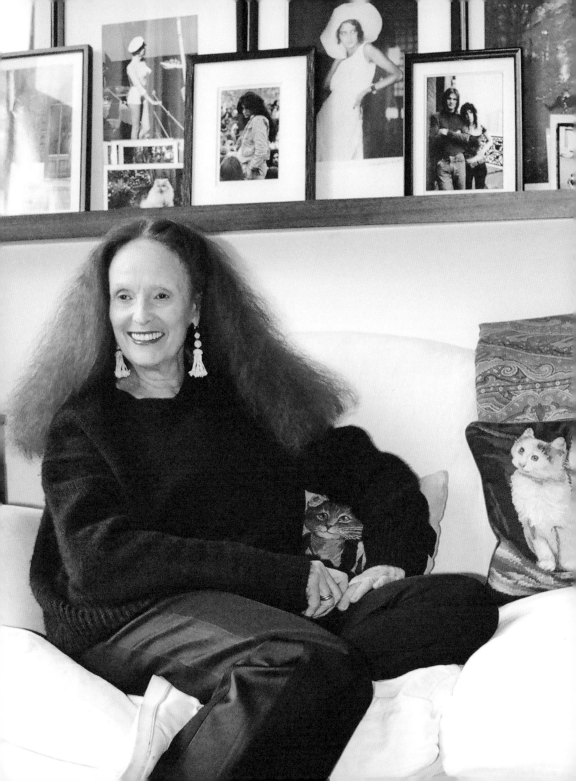

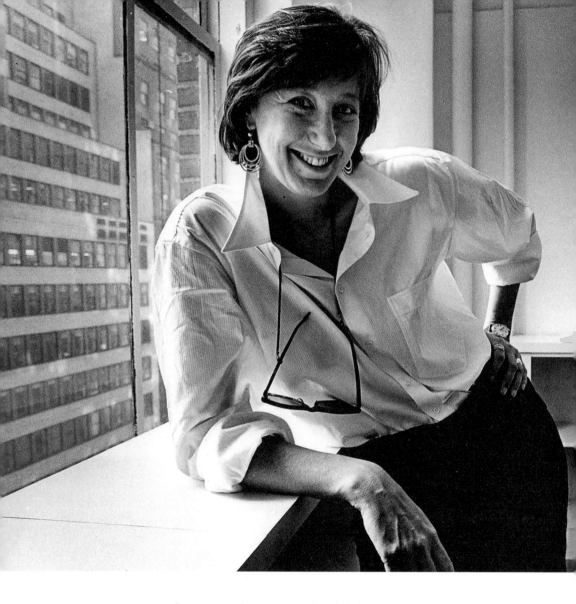

'I wanted everything to feel like a second skin,
with nothing pulling at you as you moved. It
was a new kind of classicism – like a man's
wardrobe, but tailored for a strong woman.'

DONNA KARAN

USA, born 1948

L et's spin back to 1985, when Donna Karan launched her own brand, focusing on the needs of the working woman with her Seven Easy Pieces. This capsule wardrobe was based on the 'body', an all-in-one jersey top that fastened with press studs under the gusset (making going to the lavatory a whole new experience) and created a smooth, stream-lined silhouette. The body was designed to be mixed and matched with the other pieces, including a draped skirt that was flattering to anyone who didn't have a washboard-flat stomach. The system would transform the wardrobes of working women, enabling them to look both strong and feminine, rather than simply aping their male counterparts' wardrobes.

After dropping out of Parsons School of Art in New York, Karan trained with Anne Klein and then took over as creative director when the designer died. Karan had given birth to her daughter Gabby the same week, so she understood fully the demands and challenges of trying to do it all: have children *and* a high-profile career while being in fashion's limelight, where looks are everything.

In Karan's aspirational world, it seemed that if you had the right wardrobe and enough confidence,

anything was possible. In 1989 she founded a more accessible line, DKNY, which channelled the youth-ful energy of New York, as a wardrobe for her teenage daughter and her friends. In 1992 she created an ad campaign featuring a female president dressed in a double-breasted pinstriped suit. She developed a friendship with Hillary Clinton, whom she dressed in her bestselling Cold Shoulder dress, a high-necked jersey tube with cut-outs at the shoulders – Karan's favourite erogenous zone – for her first official White House dinner after Bill Clinton's inauguration as President of the United States in 1993. She sold her stake in Donna Karan in 2015 to focus on her lifestyle brand, Urban Zen, which is run as a philan-thropic exercise to raise money for and awareness of children's education, artisanal preservation and support for Haiti.

The impact of Karan's Seven Easy Pieces cannot be overstated. The mix of masculine and feminine, sensuous and practical – not to mention the camel coat, the crisp shirt, the slouchy trousers, all ingre-dients of Phoebe Philo's later success at Céline (see page 92) – provided the perfect balance for a new generation of women, like her, on the move.

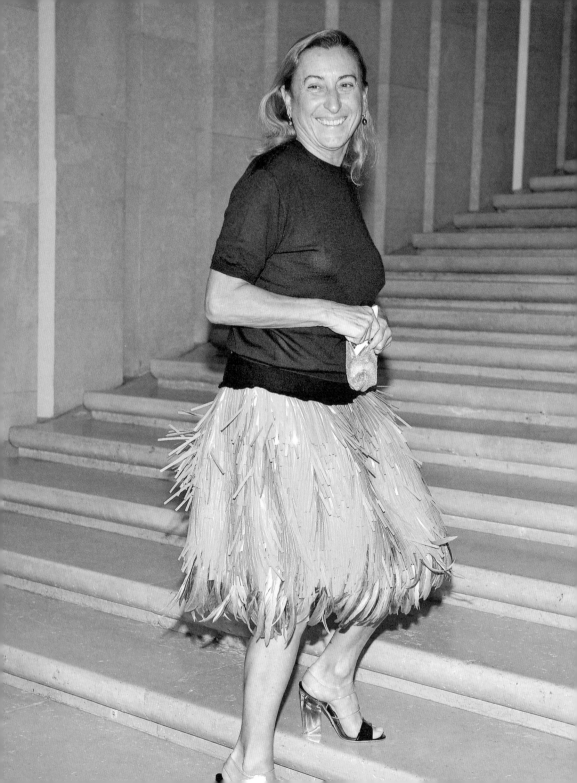

MIUCCIA PRADA

Italy, born 1949

'My best quality is my instinct.'

In 1984 Miuccia Prada revolutionized luxury fashion with a nylon rucksack. Hardly the height of chic, you might think, but this one was. In 1980s designer black, with its little triangular label inscribed 'Prada', it became symbolic of a new generation of designer shoppers for whom status was everything. Her 'It' bag (as it was to become in the 1990s) was made as a utilitarian backpack: industrial, functional and thoroughly modern, just the thing to carry to your nouvelle cuisine dinner in the latest 'designer' restaurant.

'I hated all the bags that were around. They were so formal, so lady, so traditional, so classic,' Prada said. For her, nylon was all about lightness and practicality. She was a hands-free type of woman with a busy life to lead, and a chic little backpack was her solution. Clothes – made of nylon, of course (this was a time before the world became obsessed with plastics in the ocean) – followed the bags. This was a label that would go on to create frissons of desire and become one of the most influential of the late twentieth and early twenty-first centuries.

Funnily enough, Prada studied not fashion but political science. She was a member of the Italian Communist Party in the 1970s and is often cited as a 'feminist' designer, as though it is unusual for a feminist to make fashion. But this 'feminism' often simply manifests itself as clothes that appeal to women rather than to their male admirers. Such clothes are designed not to get you a rich husband but to signify that you have money and that it's your own to do with as you like. Themselves the objects of desire, these clothes might not make you look conventionally sexy (Giorgio Armani once called them 'ugly'), but rather interesting, opinionated, a thinker.

Prada is a designer to whom the fashion world always looks for a direction, an idea, a feeling for what's next. One of her early collections was described as *The Flintstones* meets *The Jetsons*, and she took it as a compliment. She has very wide taste, and that tends to make everyone else rethink their own ideas of what is tasteful or not. She might mix a 1970s chunky knit with brown leather and a canary-yellow beaded skirt trimmed with blue and white ostrich feathers. It's all very wrong, but, once it's been through the cliché-busting, contrarian Prada filter, it's what everyone wants to wear.

PHOEBE PHILO

France, born 1973

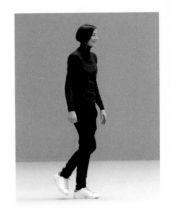

'The chicest thing is when you don't exist on Google.'

A lot has been written about Phoebe Philo, the designer credited with reinventing the modern woman's wardrobe during her time at Chloé and then Céline, but Philo herself prefers not to say much. She's never been interested in being the celebrity designer, a 'face'; she is a quieter, more instinctive designer who is not particularly interested in analyzing what she does or telling the world what she's having for breakfast.

That Philo has taken career breaks to have her children really shouldn't be remarkable, but it is at her level in the fashion industry. She has always played by her own rules, and has gained respect for that. Her clothes speak for themselves – assured, confident, empowering, strong – and are, for many women, valuable tools to express who they are in a way that keeps an air of glamour and femininity while not sexualizing, fetishizing or underplaying them in any way. The quality and craftsmanship have always justified the expense, and these clothes were designed to stand the test of time. Not surprisingly, when Philo announced in 2017 that she was leaving her job at Céline, it was a blow for her loyal customers. Although most had never met her, they felt a personal relationship – even a friendship

– with the designer who seemed so closely in tune with their needs. The fashion critic Cathy Horyn described her departure from Céline as 'a watershed moment'.

Philo, who started out as Stella McCartney's partner in crime at Chloé, has an innate sense of what is cool and, most importantly, an uncanny connection with what women want a season before they realize it themselves. She used an 80-year-old Joan Didion in her Spring/Summer 2015 advertising campaign, and you believed that Didion would – and no doubt does – choose to wear Céline. Philo plays nobody's game but her own, and has that most elusive of qualities, integrity.

Philo's impact on the wardrobes of a generation of women – her own generation – has been as great as Coco Chanel's was on hers (see page 78). For that reason, it will endure beyond the designer's tenure at any one house. She is generally credited with giving women a uniform: slouchy trousers, a blouse or crisp white shirt, a camel coat and a faintly edgy statement boot, all worn with an interesting piece of jewellery. That so many women identify with this look, and use it to support themselves in their working lives, is quite a legacy.

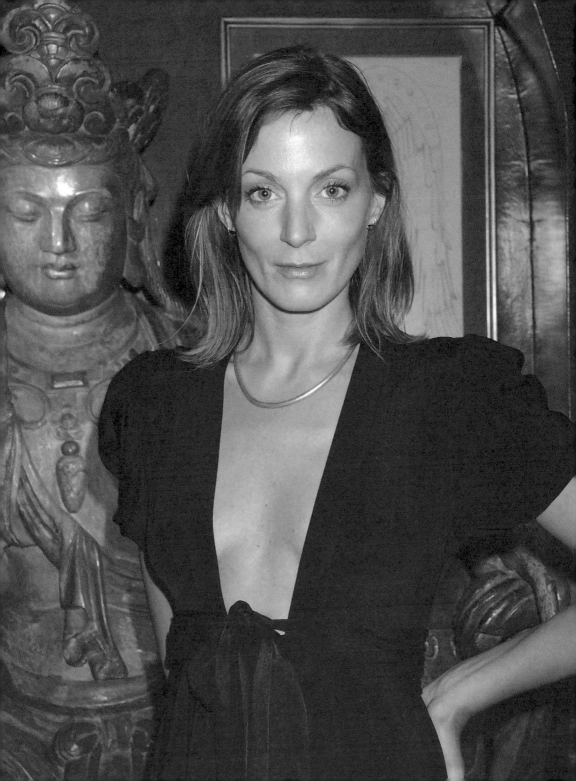

MOLLY GODDARD

UK, born 1988

'My main thing is I like women to be comfortable.'

According to Lynn Yaeger in *Vogue*, Molly Goddard's frothy, oversized net dresses in a range of sometimes teeth-jarring colours have 'a transgressive current rumbling underneath all the frothy folderol [and] a rebellious spirit that is as feminist as it is feminine.'

It's transgressive, maybe, but there's nothing threatening about a Goddard smock. Her BA collection was based on clothes from her childhood, blown up to adult size on the photocopier. She does not infantilize women, however: when Rihanna wears her dresses (she has several), she looks anything but childlike and innocent. There's something extreme about the sheer volume of tulle, the cloud of electric colour that envelops the wearer. Goddard says she would like her granny to wear her clothes, and indeed there's a feeling that you could be any size, shape, age or even gender and be happy in one of her pieces. Her collaboration with the photographer Tim Walker resulted in *Patty* (named after her pet guinea pig), a book of portraits of her friends wearing pieces from her archive.

Goddard's first show, in 2013, was actually a party. In a church. Her boyfriend Thomas Shickle had encouraged her to do it, and she roped in her sister Alice, a stylist, and her mother to help with the staging. They gave Goddard's smocks to friends to put on over what they were already wearing. That's the thing about Goddard: she makes sheer party dresses that are designed to be worn for the everyday, over jeans and trainers or whatever you happen to be wearing. They are the grown-up equivalent of the nursery dressing-up box, when you got to wear a princess dress for the afternoon. It's a fantasy, and you can wear it with as much irony and knowingness as you like. They are not particularly designed to be worn over a perfect body with sexy underwear.

Goddard has said she likes that moment when 'you're feeling grown up in whatever you were wearing, but that slight awkwardness of being maybe a bit too dressed up for your age or your mentality'. She likes things to be clunky around the edges – too big, too small, not quite right. Goddard herself exudes something of a modern-day Alice in Wonderland, with her waist-length strawberry-blonde fringed hair and natural, freckled face. She is emblematic of a generation of women who don't overthink their clothes or take fashion too seriously, but like to make a bit of an entrance without looking as though they've tried too hard.

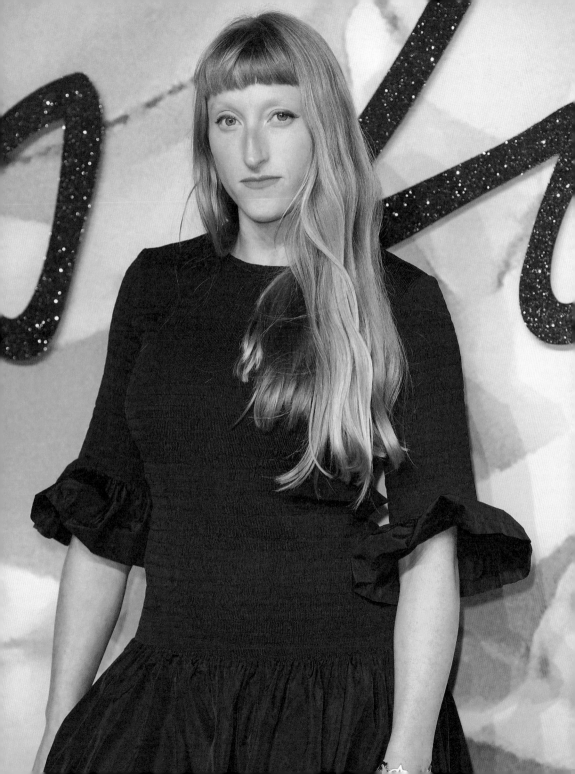

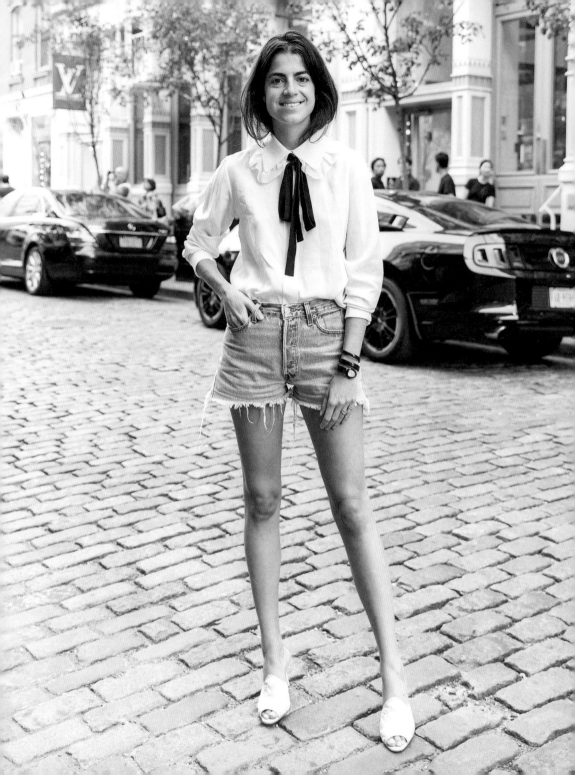

LEANDRA MEDINE

USA, born 1988

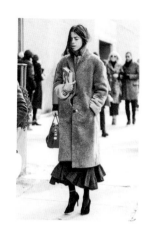

'If it feels wrong, it probably looks right.'

An interest in fashion doesn't minimize one's intellect. That's the simple premise for Leandra Medine's extraordinarily influential online magazine, *Man Repeller,* which she describes as 'a judgement free zone that allows you to be who you are, pants unbuttoned and all'. In 2010, when she started her style blog about trends that women love and men hate, she wanted to write about fashion in a way that was humorous, intelligent and personal. While she could easily have become a thorn in the side of the industry, her enthusiasm is infectious. She wants *Man Repeller* to be your older sister's kind friend (because your older sister probably isn't so kind, at least not to you).

Born Leandra Medine Cohen, Medine is a true Manhattanite. She went to school on the Upper East Side and started online writing while studying journalism at the New School. Her first blog, *Boogers and Bagels,* evolved into *Man Repeller* in 2010. Her irreverent, witty take on fashion was inspired by a session in the fitting rooms of Topshop, when her friend told her she didn't have a boyfriend because she didn't dress for men.

What we love about Medine is her messy hair, the fact that she looks as though she was up late and then slept in, her Sandra Bernhard dry-as-a-bone sense of humour and the fact that ultimately, even though it now pays her bills, she takes the fashion industry with a good pinch of salt. It helps that she's tall and willowy and can wear a beaten-up pair of jeans rolled halfway up her legs with a pair of calf-length socks, ankle boots and a ragged old cardigan and still have the street-style snappers chasing her down the road. Even when she's dressing up for an event, she will wear trousers when everyone else is in a skirt and heels – and somehow everyone else will look wrong. Medine confesses to suffering from low self-esteem, but in a world filled with insecurity, she makes you feel you are not alone. She is a confidence boost when you are feeling a little unsure of yourself, the girlfriend you wished you had.

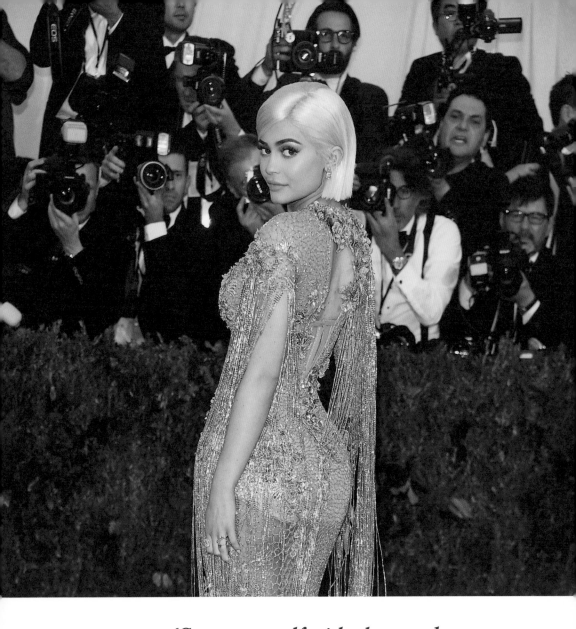

'Carry yourself with class and
dignity and don't let ANYONE
determine your future.'

KYLIE JENNER

USA, born 1997

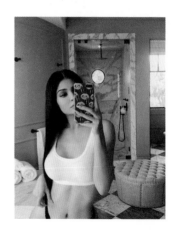

K ylie Jenner needs no introduction. She was thrust into the limelight at the age of nine as part of the most famous, most oversharing family in the history of mankind. Love them or loathe them, there's no escaping the Kardashians. Jenner is the ultimate BFF whose greatest talent is not her ability to shape her brows (her personal make-up artist does that for her), change outfits every half-hour or sell you the shade of lipstick she is wearing by the tens of thousands. No, what she is really, really good at is making you feel that you are part of her life.

Jenner's is in the Top 10 most popular Instagram feeds, with more than 115 million followers. Everything she does is shared, scrutinized – and imitated. When the #KylieJennerChallenge (which involved sucking your lips inside a glass bottle or shot glass to cause swelling similar to her overblown lips) turned into the #KylieJennerChallengeGoneWrong, with pictures of teens and their bruised and misshapen lips, Jenner made a statement: 'I'm not here to try & encourage people/young girls to look like me or to think this is the way they should look.'

Jenner says her only passion is make-up (although that was before the birth of her daughter Stormi

Webster in February 2018). It's not surprising when you consider that she grew up in a household where hair and make-up are a major part of daily life. By the age of 12 she was an expert in mascara and lip liner, and she's used her knowledge to great effect. She launched her super-brand, Kylie Cosmetics, in November 2015, with its signature dripping lips icon. The first three products – three shades of lipstick – sold out within seconds of her promoting them online, and the brand is predicted to reach $1 billion in sales by 2022.

Considering she was born into a life of extreme privilege, wealth and preordained fame, Jenner is no slouch. She admits that the pressure of feeding her social-media life – keeping those hyper-real lips pumped up, the wigs washed and ready to go, the make-up flawless, the clothes fitting to a nano-stitch of her Jessica-Rabbit-on-steroids curves – is relentless, but she has a close-knit team to support her every move.

The reality is that Jenner's influence is not something she can control. Whether she continues to be the world's BFF remains to be seen, but she has a few more years before Stormi (139,000 followers and counting) steals the limelight.

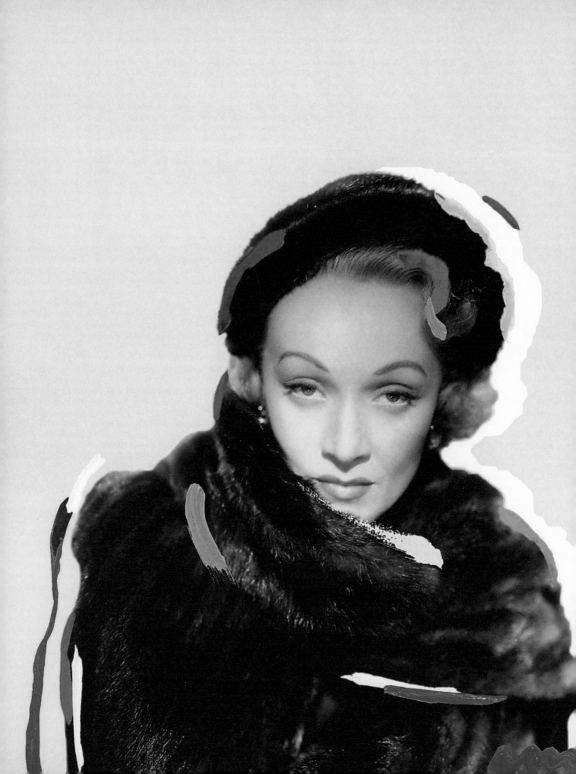

Silver-Screen Dreams

These are the women who paved the way for many others to look, behave and shine like the superstars they are. Sure, they all had a certain amount of sex appeal – to both men and women – but they were also strong characters, and many led lives that were as extraordinary off-screen as they were on it. They used their image to project who they were and what they stood for. They were goddesses in every sense, and the inspiration for generations of women after them.

MARLENE DIETRICH

Germany, 1901–1992

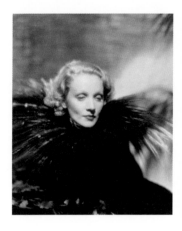

'I am at heart a gentleman.'

It is impossible to overstate the extraordinary influence of Marlene Dietrich. From her famous heavily hooded bedroom eyes, her gender-fluid top hat and tails, and the seductively limited range of her husky singing voice to the glamorous image she presented to her public both on- and off-screen, she was the ultimate celluloid star.

Dietrich was raised in Berlin at the beginning of the twentieth century, and found her way into the theatre. In 1930 she played the cabaret singer Lola Lola in the Paramount film *The Blue Angel*, and her brooding, subversive, highly sexualized image was burned into the subconscious of a generation. She moved to America shortly afterwards, and when the Nazi regime attempted to persuade her to return to Germany, she refused. She helped to finance refugees escaping from Nazi Germany in the late 1930s, and made propaganda recordings to boost the morale of the Allied soldiers. 'Lili Marleen' became her signature tune as she spent the war years performing to the troops. She was awarded the Legion of Honour in France, and in 2002 was made an honorary citizen of Berlin.

Dietrich was an alpha female in every way, and the characters she played were always fiercely independent. She married only once, but had an impressive list of lovers (from James Stewart to John F. Kennedy), as well as some pretty fabulous women, whom she referred to as the 'Sewing Circle'. Her penchant for wearing men's suits – a look and confidence later adopted by Madonna (see page 51) – was not so much a fashion statement as a proud symbol of her bisexuality. Suzanne Vega's song 'Marlene on the Wall' of 1986 was inspired by Dietrich's erotic charms.

Dietrich's don't-mess-with-me attitude shone through whether she was wearing a shimmering, beaded, figure-hugging gown, a lacy negligee and suspenders, or a shirt and tie. The male-dominated film world of the era might explain why some of the more strident female stars of the 1930s opted to wear trousers when they were off duty. 'Women's clothes take too much time – it is exhausting, shopping for them,' said Dietrich. 'Men's clothes do not change. I can wear them as long as I like.'

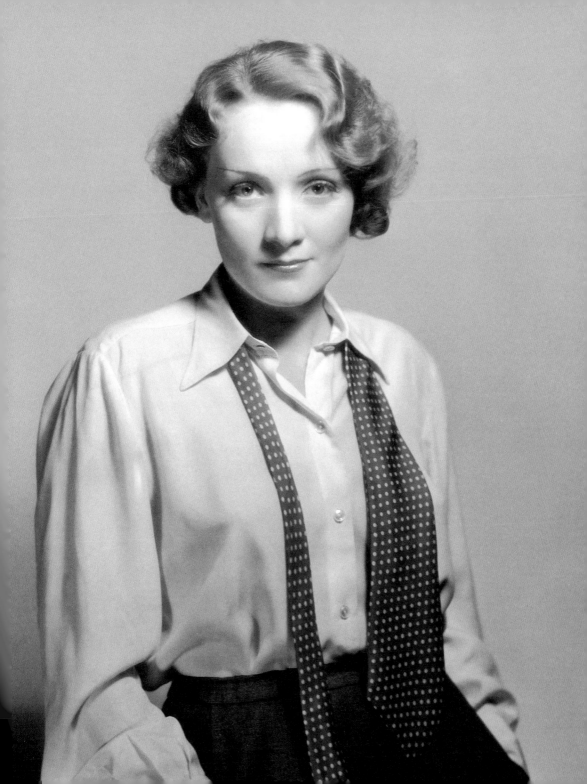

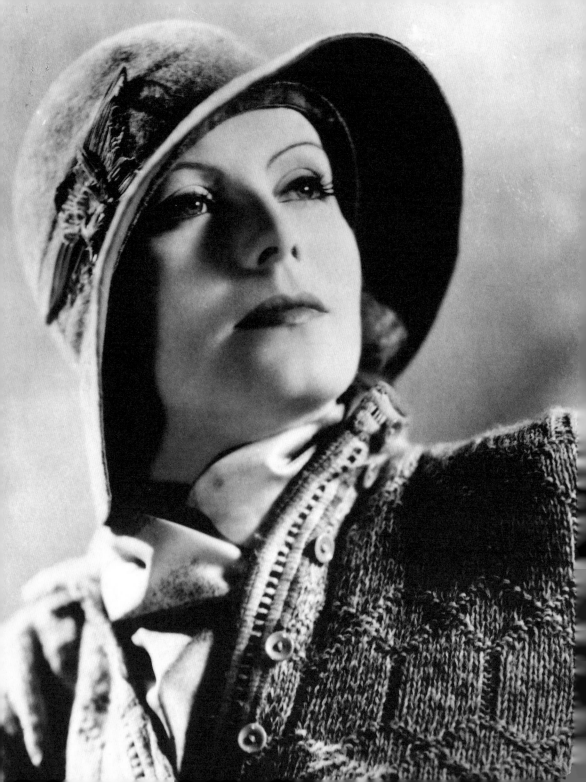

GRETA GARBO

Sweden, 1905–1990

'I like to live simply ... dress simply.'

She was a solitary soul, an independent spirit who was not interested in being part of the crowd. And Greta Garbo had a style all her own, too. Garbo, as she quickly became known, had a penchant for a statement hat, whether a slouchy cloche pulled down over her straight hair, a cool beret (the level of cool that Dior's Maria Grazia Chiuri could only dream of achieving when she introduced the beret for 2017) or a fabulously floppy, wide-brimmed fedora to frame one of the most exquisite faces ever to grace the silver screen.

Garbo arrived in Hollywood from Stockholm in 1925 at the age of 19. Famous for her aloofness, she simply shrugged and said she would return to Sweden when MGM refused to give her more money. The attitude paid off, and her appeal at the box office gave the studio no choice but to pay up.

Garbo quickly gained a reputation for not joining the Hollywood gatherings and society parties, preferring to go for walks on the beach. The roles she played, from Queen Christina to Mata Hari, tended to reflect that seriousness and sense of independence. In *Grand Hotel* (1932) she utters the immortal line, 'I want to be alone.' She made it all right for women to want their own space, to revel in their own melancholy.

Garbo's personal style was pared-down and simple. At the time she was even considered frumpy, as though she wanted to downplay her dazzling beauty. Such simplicity was ahead of its time, and she was the original Scandi style icon: modern, classic, understated. Consider her wardrobe (by the costume designer Adrian, but inspired by her own easy style) for *The Single Standard* in 1929: white trousers, casual Henley shirt and white tennis shoes. She was the queen of the smoky eye, soft charcoal-grey weighing down the lids of her eyes, her thick eyelashes so long they looked false. Whatever she wore, from her hairstyle to her mannish trousers and mysterious trench coats, became all the rage. Nearly 40 years later Faye Dunaway borrowed from her cool simplicity for her role in *Bonnie & Clyde* (1967). And Garbo's style has never really looked old.

Garbo stopped making films in 1941, at the age of 35, sensing that her integrity as an actor was in jeopardy. She knew that less is more. Garbo really is eternal.

KATHARINE HEPBURN

USA, 1907–2003

'I liked to look as if I didn't give a damn.'

A heroine for all women who don't like to play the game, and who dress to please themselves and no one else, Katharine Hepburn was headstrong, fearless and sublimely elegant – especially in a trouser suit. 'We're all in a pretty serious spot when the original bag lady wins a prize for the way she dresses,' she quipped when she was given the Lifetime Achievement Award by the Council of Fashion Designers of America in 1986.

At ten, a steadfast Kate Hepburn cut her hair short, wore boys' clothes and called herself Jimmy. She said she wanted to be a boy because her brothers had all the fun. She was encouraged to be independent by her radical parents (her mother was educated at university at a time when few women were, her father a surgeon who led on sexual hygiene). The fearless tomboy grew up a feisty, beautiful, freethinking woman driven by a desire to act – and to be famous. When she moved to New York in the late 1920s, she was still dressing in scuffed-up old boys' clothes, without make-up. She was a novelty, and that is what set her apart.

When Hepburn moved to Hollywood, she was cast as a strong-willed daughter and became an instant star. She was unlike any other female actor of the time: boyish, athletic, strident and with a directness that made you sit up in your cinema seat and take notice. Unlike Marlene Dietrich and Greta Garbo (see pages 102 and 105), who conformed to some kind of male lesbian fantasy, Hepburn's masculine style was about ease of movement and equality.

In the world of #MeToo and the gender pay gap scandal, Hepburn seems a pioneer. She demanded more pay than her peers; she drove around Hollywood in her own station wagon and turned up at the studio in denim overalls, looking more like a mechanic than a sex siren. She said she liked trousers because they looked better with flat shoes. She wanted to look as though there was more interesting stuff going on in her life than staring into a mirror doing her make-up and trying on silk dresses. It was about showing brains as well as beauty, but she couldn't escape her own innate style. Above all, Hepburn stood for simplicity. Nobody has ever looked more at ease in her own skin, wearing a perfect white cotton shirt and a cool pair of slacks.

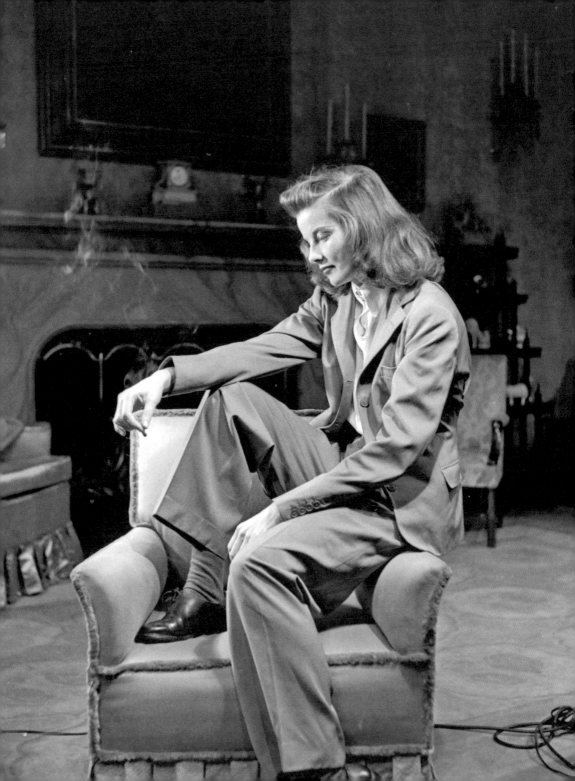

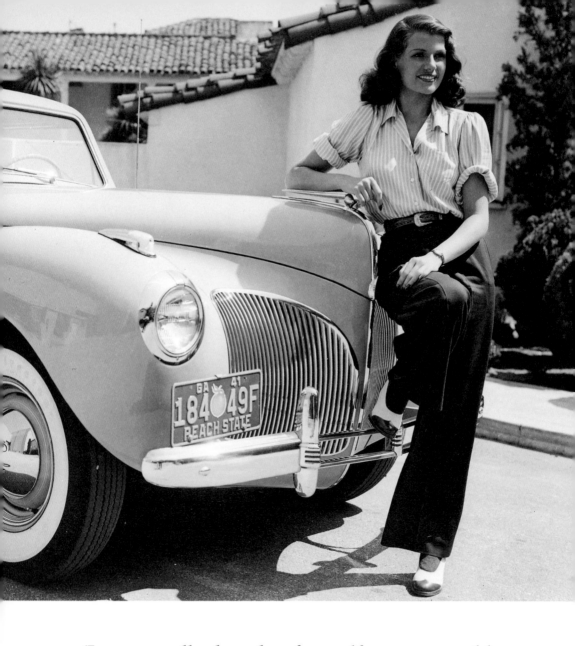

'I never really thought of myself as a sex goddess:
I felt I was more a comedian who could dance.'

RITA HAYWORTH

USA, 1918–1987

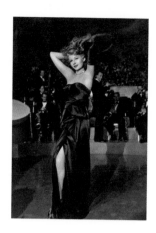

The transformation from Margarita Carmen Cansino, daughter of two dancers, to Rita Hayworth, Hollywood's most glamorous seductress, is stark. Publicity pictures of the aspiring starlet in 1940 show a beautiful young woman with a centre parting and shiny black hair. Later images show a dramatic change. Hayworth's hairline was altered with electrolysis (a Hollywood studio fetish at the time) and her hair dyed red and waved into one of her most famous features.

It wasn't just the hairline that had proved too 'Latin' for the studio bosses. Cansino became Hayworth (a version of her Irish-English mother's maiden name). In her natural incarnation, she was cast as an Egyptian beauty in *Charlie Chan in Egypt* (1935), and with her olive skin and black hair she was fair game for the culturally blind, indiscriminate Hollywood 'world' casting couch. But as red-headed Rita Hayworth, she became a huge star.

A childhood spent dancing professionally in Tijuana, Mexico (her abusive father started teaching her when she was four), meant she was a match for Fred Astaire and Gene Kelly, both of whom she partnered. She performed one of the most seductive dances ever as the femme fatale Gilda in Charles

Vidor's film of that name (1946). The press called her 'the Love Goddess', and she was every GI's sweetheart during World War II. The atomic bomb that America dropped as a test on Bikini Atoll in 1946 was named Gilda. Hayworth, who married five times in total – all disastrous – was Hollywood's first princess, marrying Prince Aly Khan in 1949. (Her first marriage, at 18, had been to her 41-year-old manager, who saw her as an investment and encouraged her to sleep with anyone who might further her career.)

However manufactured her glamour was (and she favoured comfortable, practical clothes in real life), Hayworth was a great influence on how women aspired to dress. The wardrobe designed for Gilda by Jean Louis had a huge budget, but for war-weary audiences it was worth every penny. She had 'the Look' of the decade, from her long, red, wavy hair to her full-length satin gloves. The famous black satin strapless gown that seemed to be miraculously moulded to her body however she moved has become one of the most copied dresses, a perennial red-carpet design. To ensure it did not malfunction, there was a harness inside it and the bra top was made of plastic, designed not to move. It can't have been comfortable, but Hayworth makes it look like a second skin.

LAUREN BACALL

USA, 1924–2014

'I think your whole life shows in your face and you should be proud of that.'

It was her cool swagger more than anything. That, and the matt-ness of her lipstick and those quizzically arched brows. Lauren Bacall exuded a worldly confidence that belied her total lack of it. Even when young and inexperienced – her first role was at 19 in *To Have and Have Not* (1944), in which she tells her co-star and future husband Humphrey Bogart how to whistle: 'you just put your lips together and blow' – she exuded sophisticated glamour and superior insolence. There was never any doubt that Bacall was in complete control of the situation. With those shoulder pads, how could she be anything but?

Born Betty Joan Perske, Bacall was renamed 'Lauren' by the great director Howard Hawks. Her career had been kick-started as a model in 1942, when she was introduced to Diana Vreeland (see page 36), then fashion editor of *Harper's Bazaar*. Bacall was 17, and terrified of the imposing Vreeland, who put her in front of Louise Dahl-Wolfe's camera for a test. 'I felt like a gawk,' she wrote in her memoir *By Myself and Then Some* (2005). 'Never thought I was a beauty, so I never really expected too much.'

In March 1943 Bacall was on the cover of the magazine, wearing a tailored suit with a dramatic upturned collar, a silk scarf tied around her neck by Vreeland herself, a red leather satchel on one wrist and a skullcap over her naturally wavy red hair. Seemingly unaware of the power of her beauty, she was delighted to be earning $10 an hour modelling, and, although still a teenager, she looked every bit the woman of the world. When she made the transformation from magazine star to movie star, that was her persona: cigarette-toting, wisecracking, knowingly seductive and husky-voiced. She had a way of looking at the camera with her chin down, catching the viewer in a perpetual eye lock. Warner Bros called it 'The Look', and it was mesmerizing. Bogart thought so, certainly: their love affair was electric, both on- and off-screen.

Bacall had caught Vreeland's eye not so much because of her clothes as her cool way of moving, her direct manner and far more than any woman's allotted glamour quotient. A natural beauty, she had thick eyebrows and crooked teeth, which she insisted shouldn't be changed. She refused to be moulded by the studio into something she was not. She's a standard-bearer for confident, sexy, unashamedly alluring women everywhere; the fact that she was trembling inside makes her all the more appealing.

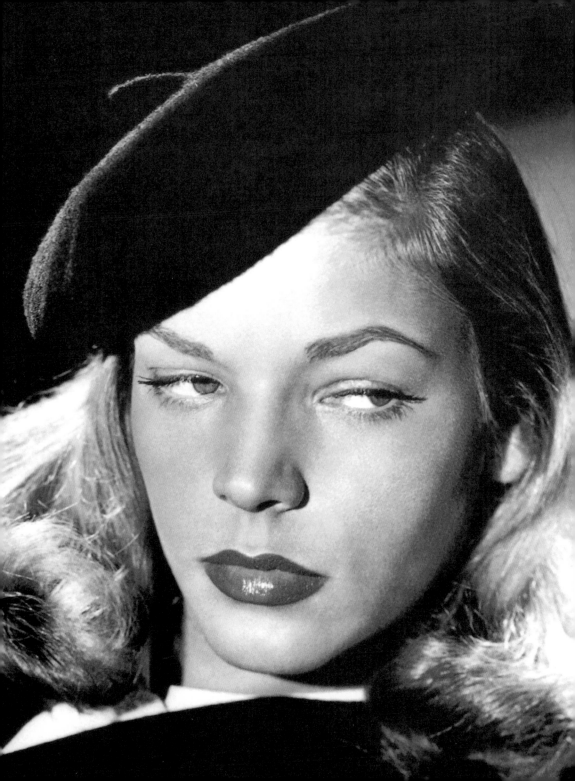

MARILYN MONROE

USA, 1926–1962

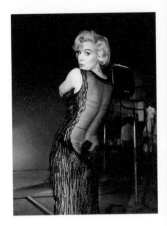

'Give a girl the right pair of shoes and she'll conquer the world.'

The fact that Marilyn Monroe was turned down by Paramount before being signed by 20th Century Fox will give hope to anyone who has ever been rejected for anything. But her story is one of endless determination and dogged perseverance. Her first film roles in the late 1940s amounted to little more than a few lines between them, but she was determined to escape from the boredom of being a housewife (she had married at 16 to avoid being sent back to an orphanage after a childhood spent in care and abusive foster homes). Success was a long time coming, but she didn't give up.

Monroe was defined by her sexuality, which she used to further her own success and also fought against. She was gloriously funny, sexy, impossibly beautiful and a camp caricature of every man's (and many women's) fantasy. She married Joe DiMaggio, the baseball star, and Arthur Miller, the playwright. She veered from voluptuous physicality to a deep craving to be taken seriously as an actor and an intelligent human being, but few in Hollywood were able to go beyond treating her as the ultimate dumb blonde. She spent her career being patronized, celebrated for her beauty and her extraordinary figure, and little else. It is hardly surprising that she suffered from depression and addiction to drugs and alcohol. The pressure of being her even just for one day must have been unbearable.

Of course, there's no getting away from the chemical reaction that seemed to happen when Monroe stood in front of a camera. Her role as Sugar 'Kane' Kowalczyk, the ukulele-playing singer with a penchant for saxophone players in *Some Like it Hot* (1959), features one of the most daring dresses in the history of cinema – although it is not so much the dress itself as the body inside it that makes it so extraordinary. She might as well have been naked.

In the last photographs of her, taken by the photographer Bert Stern, Monroe *is* naked, apart from a chiffon scarf. But she is utterly at ease with herself, laughing, her kohl-lined eyes slightly smudged, with shiny orange-red lips and that platinum-blonde hair.

Monroe's easy approach to her sexuality was liberating. She talked about not wearing any underwear at a time when it was fine for men to have sexual freedom, but taboo for women. She exaggerated her own considerable femininity, celebrated her curves and inspired generations of women to do the same, from Madonna to Courtney Love and even Rihanna (see pages 51, 73 and 222).

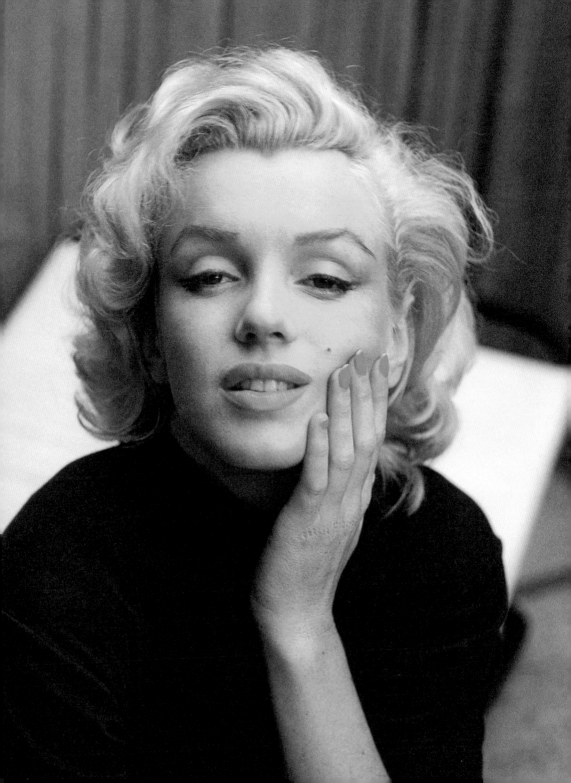

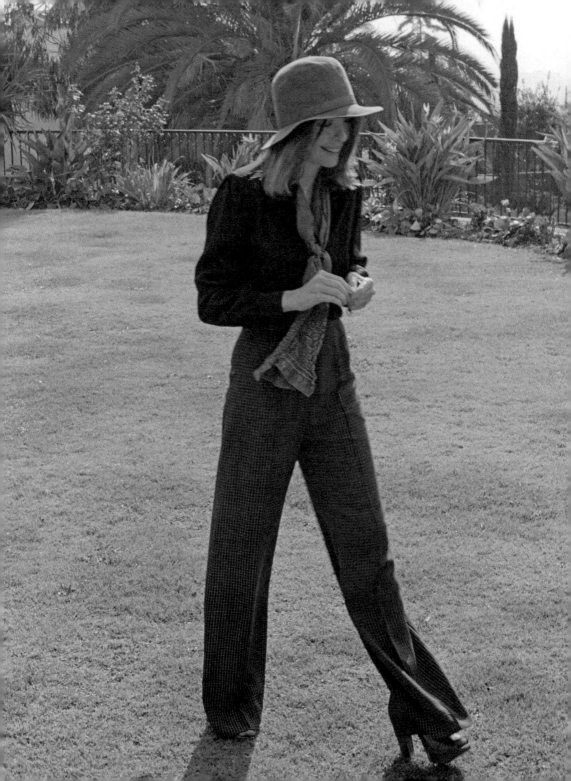

DIANE KEATON

USA, born 1946

'I stole what I wanted to wear from cool-looking women on the streets of New York.'

Diane Keaton can be credited with one of the longest-lasting, most significant fashion looks of the twentieth and twenty-first centuries. The look she created for her character in the film *Annie Hall* in 1977 is not a trend. For many women, her most famous film was a life-changing moment. Here was a woman they could really identify with: she had problems and hang-ups, and was by no means a vision of perfection. And she had a quirky, slightly eccentric way of dressing that was adopted immediately by a certain type of intelligent, bookish, left-leaning, opinionated, right-on woman.

Annie's style became a visible expression of a new freedom and independence for a generation of women keen to express their equality by playing around with men's clothes. It was a deconstructed, messed-up, softer idea of menswear. And the style belonged entirely to Keaton herself. Her original surname was Hall, and she was nicknamed Annie. Ralph Lauren is often credited with creating the wardrobe for the film, but, although Keaton was a customer and some of his clothes were in the film, the designer himself says the style was all hers. They shared a love of oversized slouchy jackets, waistcoats and cowboy boots. The costume designer Ruth Morley thought some of Keaton's kooky combinations went too far, but Keaton's director and co-star, Woody Allen, insisted that she be allowed to choose what to wear. The bowler hat she wore had been borrowed from a fellow actor on the set of another, most unlikely film, *The Godfather* (1972), in which Keaton played Michael Corleone's wife, Kay.

It's this authenticity that shines through and makes Annie's character so convincing. Keaton says she borrowed from the women she saw in SoHo in the mid-1970s; they, in turn, were being inspired by Patti Smith (see page 66). Keaton also admires the style of Marlene Dietrich and Katharine Hepburn (see pages 102 and 106), both of whom experimented with men's clothing.

That Keaton's look often appears thrown together, with pieces layered haphazardly, is all part of her saying she has a busy, multifaceted life and does not have time to blow-dry her hair and get her nails done. It's a look and an attitude that are very relevant today, and Keaton herself has never tired of either.

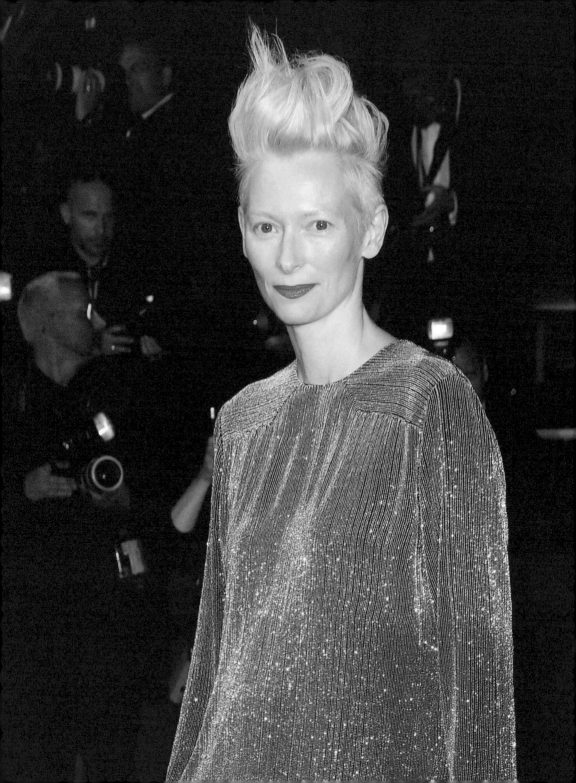

TILDA SWINTON

UK, born 1960

'I would rather be handsome ... for an hour than pretty for a week.'

Who doesn't love Tilda Swinton? She could fit into many of the chapters in this book, but most of us know her through the cinema screen, where she has held her own, seemingly supernaturally transcending any kind of ageing process, for more than 30 years.

You may know Swinton as the White Witch in the Narnia films of the early 2000s, or as David Bowie's wife and doppelgänger in his video for 'The Stars (Are Out Tonight)' (2013). She may have changed your life – at least, whom you could or couldn't fall in love with – in the adaptation of Virginia Woolf's *Orlando* (1992). It seems almost impossible that she made her film debut in 1986, in the cult director Derek Jarman's *Caravaggio*. Since then she has become shorthand for 'art house'. When she played a 3,000-year-old ethereally beautiful, bloodless vampire in *Only Lovers Left Alive* (2013), you had to pinch yourself; maybe she really was immortal, after all.

In 1995, when Swinton spent a week apparently asleep in a glass casket as an art exhibit, people queued to look at her, a study in stillness and enviable bones. Patti Smith (see page 66) – herself the queen of androgyny – has called her 'both princess and prince', and the film director Wes Anderson described her as 'almost the colour of a cloud'. On-screen, she has been dressed by everyone from Dior (the dreamiest of all wardrobes in *A Bigger Splash*, 2015) to Raf Simons (*I Am Love*, 2009), and her clothes are always an important part of her characters. Off-screen, she is more interested in the people who design them than in the clothes themselves. The designers tend to become her friends.

Needless to say, Swinton looks suitably Tilda-ish whether she is wearing a Pringle of Scotland sweater (she was an ambassador for the brand) or a Chanel tweed suit (she was the face of the label's 'Paris-Edimbourg' collection in 2012). At home in Nairn in the Scottish Highlands, she favours boys' shirts, long-suffering jerseys and Wellington boots.

When the Dutch designers Viktor & Rolf cast Swinton in their Autumn 2003 'One Woman Show', it was the ultimate accolade. Her cropped, strawberry-blonde hair shaven asymmetrically, she opened the show dressed in a slouchy trouser suit with exaggerated shirt and tie in perfect disarray. She was followed by a small army of lookalikes, among them stars in their own right including her fellow Scottish aristocrat Stella Tennant (see page 203), hair dyed orange in homage, skin the same translucent glow, swagger almost as grand.

LUPITA NYONG'O

Mexico, born 1983

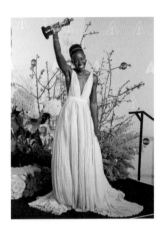

'Personally, I don't ever want to depend on make-up to feel beautiful.'

I defy anyone to watch Lupita Nyong'o's Oscar acceptance speech for Best Supporting Actress in 2014, for her role in her first ever feature film, *12 Years a Slave*, without a huge grin and tears in their eyes. There she was, dressed in an ice-blue sunray pleat dress that would have made Elizabeth Taylor proud (see page 168), an elegant band of under-stated diamonds around her hair, making a speech that was both emotional and eloquent. The dress was made by Prada, in collaboration with Nyong'o and her stylist, Micaela Erlanger, who managed to capture both Nyong'o's purity and modernity and a touch of old-school Hollywood glamour. The actor said the shade of blue reminded her of her home in Nairobi, Kenya.

Born in Mexico City but raised in Nairobi, Nyong'o has said that, although 'the history of Hollywood did not look like me,' she realized she too could have a career in the film industry when, as a child, she saw Whoopi Goldberg in *The Color Purple* (1985). The roles she carefully picks for herself, from Nakia in *Black Panther* (2018) and Nakku Harriet in *Queen of Katwe* (2016) to Patsey in *12 Years a Slave*, show an actor with a strong sense of who she is, how she can best use her talent, and her own versatility.

Nyong'o's great style icons include the Sudanese model Alek Wek, the first African model she saw on the cover of a magazine and in fashion shows. Nyong'o herself has great style. You always feel as though she believes in what she is wearing and likes experimenting with make-up. She is extremely versatile and can wear almost anything, from pastel-coloured classics to a wide variety of glorious outfits with matching colourful turbans and headwraps.

Nyong'o's op-ed for the *New York Times* in 2017, 'Speaking Out about Harvey Weinstein', gives a frank account of her encounters with the film director, which, coupled with her subsequent refusal to work on any of his films, shows her great integrity. She was admirably outspoken, too, when a photographer airbrushed her hair from the cover of *Grazia* magazine, resulting in the hashtag #DontTouchMyHair going viral.

As an extraordinary acting talent and inspiring role model, Nyong'o is the dreamiest silver-screen dream for the modern age. Intelligent, charismatic, beautiful and luminous, she is a true star.

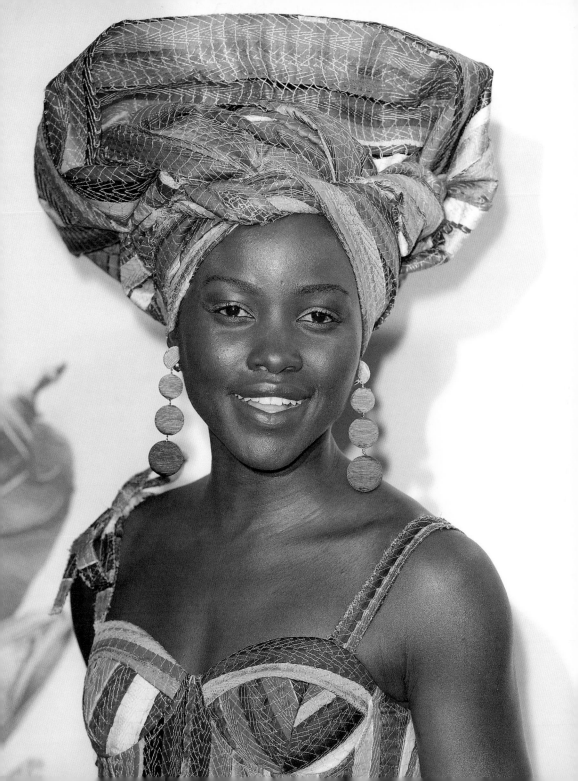

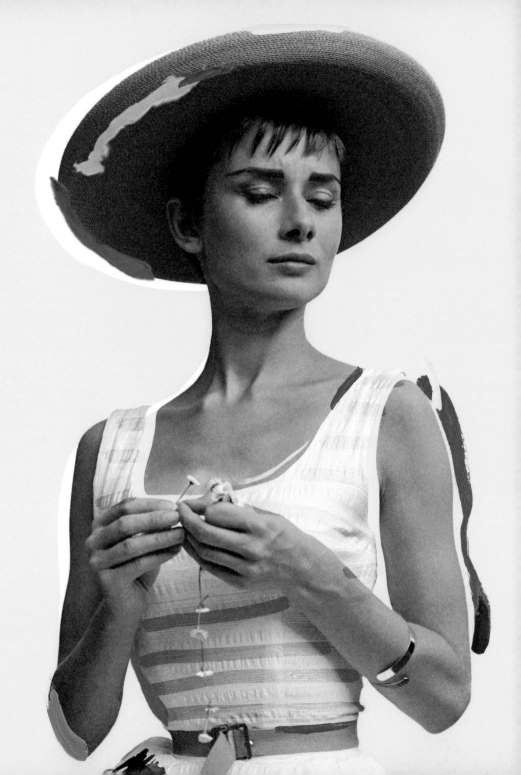

The 'It' Girls

'It' girls define a moment, somehow distilling a mood or attitude into a look and style that make time stand still forever. They have an inner spirit that spills out into everything they do. Many have a purity and intensity that are impossible to replicate – but there's no harm in trying.

AUDREY HEPBURN

Belgium, 1929–1993

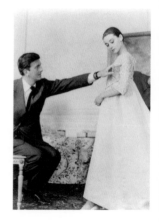

Audrey Hepburn is one of the most instantly recognizable women of the twentieth century, the ultimate gamine with her impish smile and twinkly eyes. But it is hard to separate her from Holly Golightly, the character she played in *Breakfast at Tiffany's* (1961). With a little help from her friend Hubert de Givenchy, she created a style icon in a very easily decoded uniform: little black dress, sunglasses, several strands of pearls, black elbow-length gloves, ballet pumps, cigarette holder and neat chignon. She had such universal appeal partly because of the look's simplicity and accessibility.

Hepburn's meteoric rise to stardom owed a great deal to her natural, sweet temperament. She had been spotted by the novelist Colette to play Gigi on Broadway, and from there she was offered the role of a princess in her first Hollywood film, *Roman Holiday* (1953). She was unthreatening, gentle, fawn-like – and sensational in a nipped-in waist and ballet pumps. She had trained as a ballet dancer at the Rambert in London, and her petite proportions meant that clothes always looked good on her. She had a strong sense of her own style, quite the beatnik with her black polo necks, narrow black trousers and penny loafers. It's a style that has

been adopted by endless women since, from Grace Coddington and Winona Ryder (see pages 86 and 140) to Millie Bobby Brown.

Hepburn and Givenchy enjoyed one of fashion's great love affairs. She first met him when looking for clothes to wear in *Sabrina* (1954), for which he would create costumes. There followed iconic custom-made gowns for *Funny Face* (1957) and *Breakfast at Tiffany's*. He also made clothes for Hepburn to wear off-screen, so her on- and off-screen styles became interchangeable. It was one of the first fashion and celebrity partnerships, and, through Hepburn, Givenchy was able to reach a far wider audience, keen for a touch of the Hepburn magic. If they couldn't afford the clothes, they could buy L'Interdit, the fragrance he created for her in 1957. It was a very modern relationship, although it wasn't about six-figure contracts but about friendship, loyalty and a shared love of simple, clean lines. 'His are the only clothes in which I am myself,' she said.

Ultimately, though, Hepburn's look was her own. Everything about her was neat: the short, gamine haircut, the shapely, pencilled eyebrows, the perfect ballerina poise, the irresistibly warm smile. That's not something you can get from a hanger.

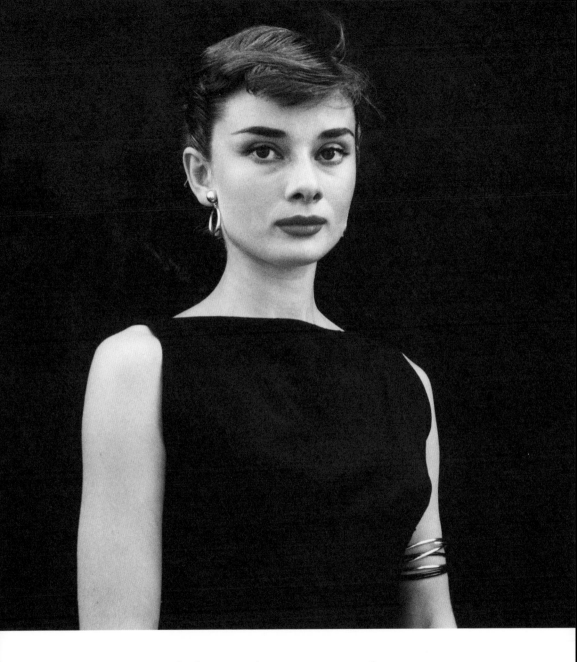

'I believe in being strong when
everything seems to be going wrong.'

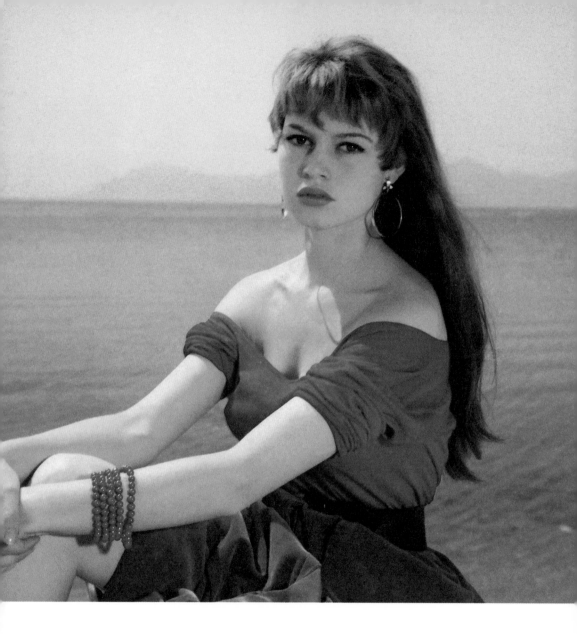

'I'm proud I created a style that
doesn't go out of fashion – because
I was never fashionable!'

BRIGITTE BARDOT

France, born 1934

In 1958 the young French film star Brigitte Bardot moved from Paris to what was then the sleepy fishing village of St-Tropez. There, the infamous star of the shocking film … *And God Created Woman* (1956; directed by her husband, Roger Vadim) hosted parties, inviting her jet-set friends to enjoy a simple life of sea-swimming and campfires. Nudity and unself-conscious sexuality were all part of this new bohemian beach scene.

Bardot, with salt in her hair, barefoot and barely bikini-bottomed, became the personification of the place. The feminist writer Simone de Beauvoir, who had watched her rise as an unashamed, empowered sex kitten, wrote: 'She goes about barefooted and turns up her nose at … all artifice. Yet her walk is lascivious and a saint would sell his soul to the devil to merely watch her dance.'

The honesty of Bardot's overt sexuality – and sensuality – was new and free. De Beauvoir argued that there was liberation and equality in the way she presented herself as a sexual being on her own terms. Her earthiness gave other women permission to flaunt their sexuality if they wished, and to be as predatory as men. It's an attitude that is commonplace today; just look at the pouting, pneumatic selfie queens on Instagram to see Bardot's legacy. With Bardot, where there was sun, sand and a sea breeze, there was sex. It was all part of nature.

Bardot brought a casualness not just to sex (her five-year marriage to Vadim fell apart because of *her* affairs, not his), but also to the way women dressed (Coco Chanel did not approve). Apparently permanently on holiday, in a bikini, a short playsuit or a pair of gingham capri pants, she created the modern Riviera style, a uniform that survives largely unchanged. Her film *The Girl in the Bikini* (1952) was seen as indecent at the time, particularly in America. She famously didn't brush her hair, unless it was to untangle knots with her fingers, and such a nonchalant attitude was shocking in the late 1950s, when women were expected to look as demure as they behaved.

Although Bardot stopped making films in 1973 to devote her life to creating an animal sanctuary, her impact on how women dressed and felt about themselves was far-reaching. It can be seen today whenever you buy a 'Bardot neckline' (which stretches from armpit to armpit), and in bikini tops and hot pants, ballet shoes and capri pants. You can even buy the texture of her sea-washed, tousled hair in a salt spray.

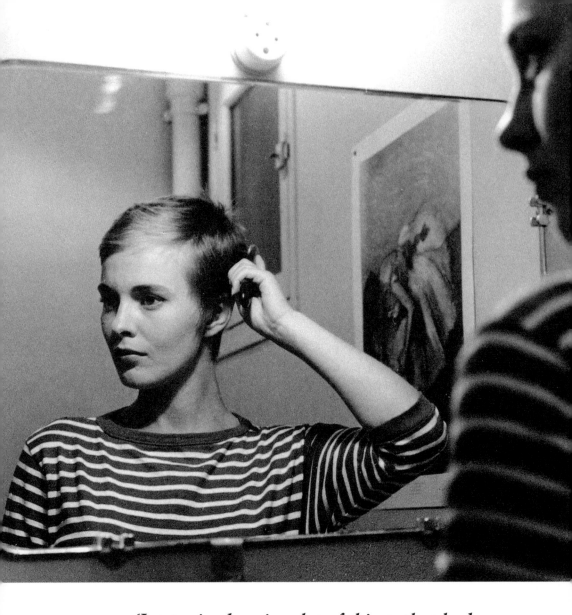

'I got mixed up in a lot of things that had
nothing to do with acting – a profession which
was coming to mean no more than getting made
up into one kind of Barbie doll or another.'

JEAN SEBERG

USA, 1938–1979

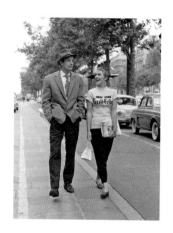

When Madonna (see page 51) made her video for 'Papa Don't Preach' in 1986, she did it in a striped boat-neck top and a short, feathery pixie haircut. It was a direct reference to one of the most outstanding style icons of all time, Jean Seberg.

The image of Seberg in Jean-Luc Godard's *À Bout de Souffle* (*Breathless*; 1960), with cropped blonde hair and wearing a *New York Herald Tribune* T-shirt with capri pants and ballet pumps, is one of the most famous in cinema history. The naturalistic style suited Seberg, and the film was an international success. Yves Saint Laurent may have elevated the basic Breton top into a Rive Gauche classic by making it into a sequinned tunic shortly afterwards, but the image of Seberg in her classic, jaunty sailor top with jeans is forever timeless – cool, natural chic at its best.

Seberg herself, a serious, intelligent woman, had moved to France after making her second film, *Bonjour Tristesse*, and marrying the French actor François Moreuil in 1958. There, she lived the dream Left Bank Parisian life, with a wardrobe full of sporty separates, in an apartment filled with abstract art,

welcoming a coterie of young artistic types. She was the proto hipster girl – arty and effortlessly cool with her natural makeup, wash-and-go hair and easy style. The French New Wave cinema critic Francois Truffaut had identified her as the genre's poster girl and her role as Patricia in *Breathless* sealed the deal.

In the 1960s she moved back to America, where she became politically active, supporting civil rights groups and the Black Panther Party, to which she donated money. Her support of the Black Panthers resulted in a programme of harassment and character assassination by the FBI, who sought to 'neutralize' her. She was blacklisted in Hollywood and her career ended (although she was in fact disenchanted by the roles she was being offered, which, she said, bordered on pornography). When she became pregnant, the FBI spread a rumour that the baby's father was the leader of the Black Panthers. She went into early labour and the baby did not survive, an experience that eventually led her to take her own life in 1979. Kristen Stewart reimagines Seberg in all her classic modernity in the political thriller *Against All Enemies* in 2019.

EDIE
SEDGWICK

USA, 1943–1971

'I made a mask out of my face because I didn't realize I was quite beautiful.'

The leotards, the tights, the boyish figure, the pixie haircut and the wide-eyed innocence gave Edie Sedgwick the look of a glamorous Peter Pan. She was Andy Warhol's dream girl, the life and soul of any party, the little rich girl gone off the rails. The two met in 1965, after Sedgwick left Harvard University and moved to New York to become a model. She quickly became a central part of the Factory, where outrageous, erratic behaviour was encouraged at all times.

Born to one of America's oldest and wealthiest families, Sedgwick had an isolated, dysfunctional childhood, spent on the family ranch in California. In Warhol's gang, she found her own family of freaks, show-offs and creative souls, and became the artist's number one Superstar. She starred in many of his films, just being herself, talking on the phone, dancing and putting on her make-up, which became her trademark. The double sets of eyelashes, endless coats of mascara and theatrical painted-on eyebrows took her up to an hour and a half.

Sedgwick was the conduit between the fashion and art worlds, which have fed off each other ever since; her role at the Factory was to be a living performance artist. She did so in a style that was to be endlessly imitated, not least after Sienna Miller played her in the film *Factory Girl* (2006): the cropped blonde hair (she sprayed her brown hair silver before bleaching it blonde), the striped jersey, tights and heels, and the hypnotic chandelier earrings that were in motion even when she was still.

Of course, it was Sedgwick's complete lack of boundaries and apparant innocence that were part of her charm. Despite her privileged background, people felt they had to protect her – up to a point. Her 15 minutes of fame didn't extend to the career she hoped for, or to any real success beyond the Warhol family. Her modelling career (she was picked up by Diana Vreeland for *Vogue* and called a 'Youthquaker', but was dropped because of her drug dependency) produced some iconic images, as Frederick Eberstadt's image here attests, but was shortlived. Her friend the fashion designer Betsey Johnson said she was 'a strange and precious flower in the Sixties and we didn't take care of her enough.'

Sedgwick's life ended in tragedy with an overdose at the age of 28. She lived hard and fast and died horribly young, defining 1960s underground New York, a moment when art, fashion, music and glamour became one and Edie Sedgwick was its shining star.

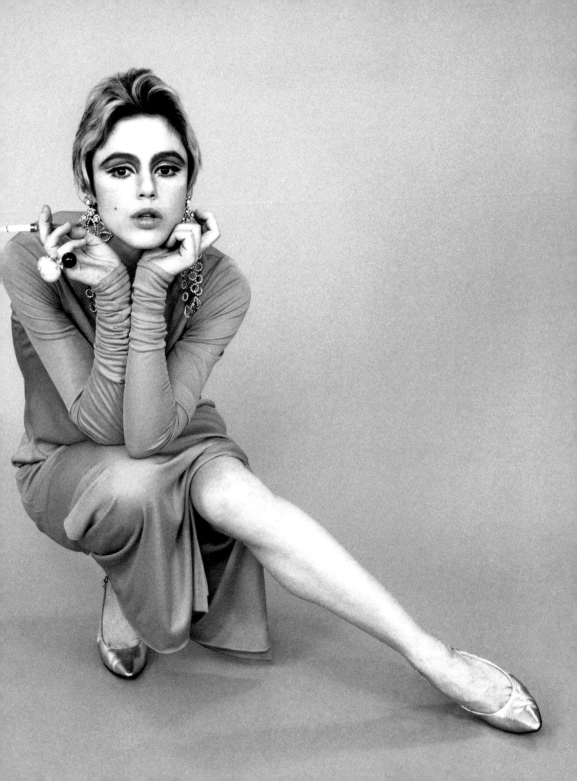

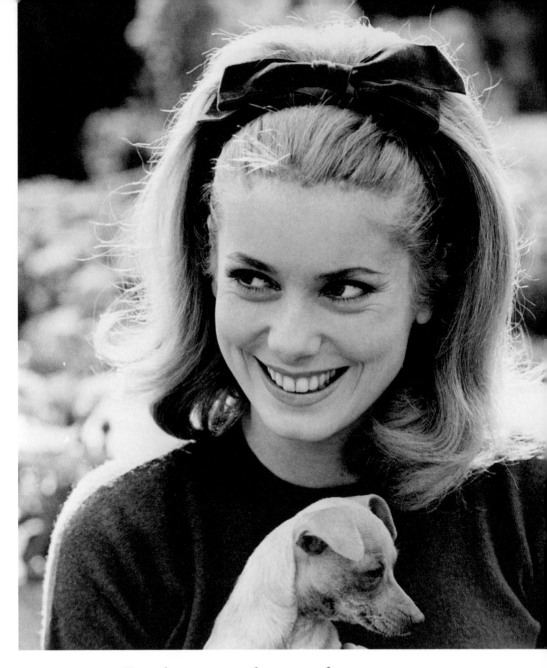

'People expect a lot more from someone
they think looks interesting.'

CATHERINE DENEUVE

France, born 1943

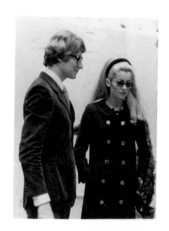

You might worry about the fate of modern-day ingénues after Catherine Deneuve was one of 100 women who signed an open letter in *Le Monde* attacking the #MeToo movement and defending men's 'right to pester'. But, for her, signing that letter was about denouncing a witch hunt against men. 'I don't excuse anything. I don't decide the guilt of these men because I am not qualified to do so. And few are … I don't like this pack mentality,' she said in her own open letter published in *Libération*, defending her position and her track record as a pioneering anti-abortion-campaigning feminist in the early 1970s.

In the 1960s, when Deneuve became a household name, the French had a more liberal attitude to sex than the rest of the world. Her breakthrough was with the jaunty, pastel-coloured musical *The Umbrellas of Cherbourg* (1964), followed the next year by Roman Polanski's psychological thriller *Repulsion*. In America, she would have been cast in endless romcoms as an elegant, cool blonde. In France – and in Italy, where she also made films – the roles were darker and more complex. *Belle de Jour* (1967), which starred Deneuve as a bored housewife who turned to prostitution to fill her empty afternoons, could not have been made anywhere but France.

What America and the rest of the world *could* understand was Deneuve's classical beauty and her European sensibility for fashion. She was queen of the red carpet and became a serious influence on how women dressed, particularly the way they wore their hair, with a slightly backcombed bouffant and a coquettish bow at the back of the head. It's a look that women still emulate today.

But Deneuve's greatest influence was as the muse of Yves Saint Laurent. Introduced to the great designer by her husband, David Bailey, Deneuve invited him to design the wardrobe for her role as Séverine in *Belle de Jour*. Saint Laurent perfectly captured the uptight, bourgeois style of the character, and the film's style has become part of the fashion lexicon. Séverine's Roger Vivier mid-heeled, square-buckled shoes sold more than 200,000 pairs following the release of the film, and are still going strong today, forever imbued with the Deneuve mystique. Saint Laurent also dressed Deneuve for 1983's cult classic vampire movie, *The Hunger*, creating another wardrobe of severe tailoring and strict, buttoned-up eroticism imbued with a dark, powerful sexuality. A little like Givenchy and Hepburn, Saint Laurent and Deneuve was a creative partnership that thrived both on- and off-screen, continuing until his death in 2008.

Now in her seventies, Deneuve continues to influence the way women dress, as well as to challenge how we think. She continues to be the perfect example of Saint Laurent's adage, 'fashion fades, style is eternal'.

FRANÇOISE HARDY

France, born 1944

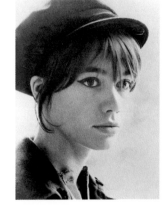

'I was always more interested in nourishing my mind than worrying about how I looked.'

How modern she looks, in a trench coat and white plastic sunglasses, clutching a camera and a book, her long dark hair and choppy 'French Girl' fringe adding a bit of sultry mystique way beyond the realms of fashion. Françoise Hardy once said that nobody would notice her if it weren't for her clothes. The archetypal Rive Gauche Sorbonne politics student-turned-singer was referring specifically to the shiny chain-metal dresses by Paco Rabanne that she wore on stage, but actually, everything about her caught the eye, even when she was at her most dressed-down. She never looked as though she had made an effort, or as though she even cared.

Hardy was too busy concentrating on her music, writing songs that went deeper than the candyfloss French pop of the 1960s girly yé-yé bands. 'Tous les garçons et les filles', the title song of her first album, recorded in 1962 when she was 18, sold more than a million copies and made it into the UK Top 40. The lyrics even became the unlikely inspiration for Rei Kawakubo's brand Comme des Garçons (see page 44). Hardy went on to record with Serge Gainsbourg, Iggy Pop and Blur.

Bob Dylan wrote a poem to Hardy and invited her to his hotel room to sing 'Just Like a Woman' and 'I Want You', but she was too star-struck to realize that he was trying to seduce her. When Brian Jones and Anita Pallenberg invited her to their home, they couldn't work out which of them she was more interested in. As it turns out, she was more taken by Mick Jagger (who described her as his ideal woman). David Bowie, too, confessed that he was in love with her: 'Every male in the world and a number of females also were,' he said.

There was clearly something about Hardy, but what was so magical about this shy, unassuming, thoughtful young singer who liked to read? The photograph of her in leathers astride a motorbike for her role in the film *Grand Prix* (1966) obviously helped. Men wanted to be with her, and women wanted to be her, dressing in her understated mix of jeans, black polo necks, classic tweeds and casual menswear. France's modernist designer Nicolas Ghesquière has used her as a style reference, describing one of his collections with a touch of 1960s military as 'a little Françoise Hardy'. She is part of French culture, embedded in the very seams of labels such as Isabel Marant and never far from the pages of *Vogue Paris*. As Alexa Chung (see page 221) says, 'what a babe'.

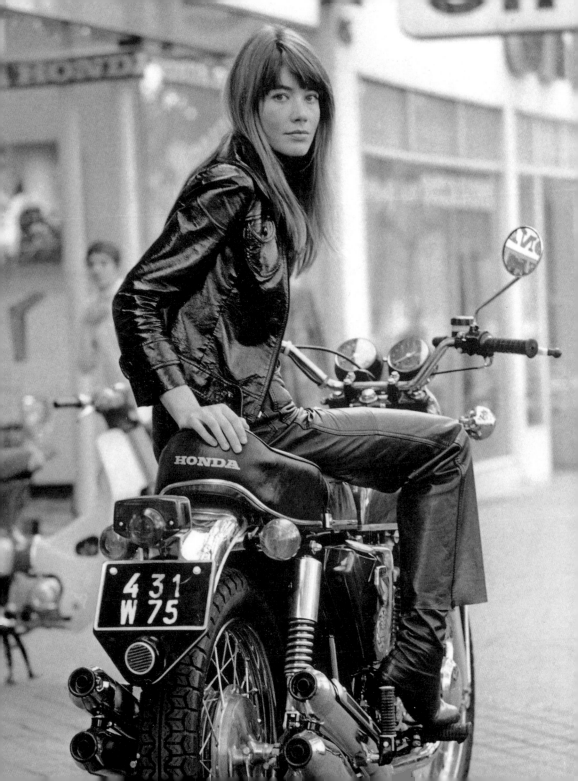

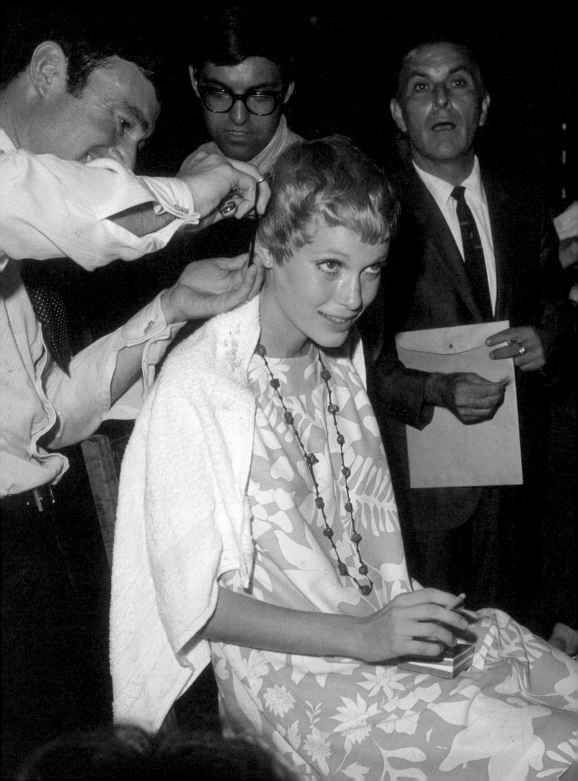

MIA FARROW

USA, born 1945

'I would rather have someone's respect than their money.'

When Mia Farrow met Frank Sinatra, in the late 1950s, she was dressed in a sheer white nightdress from the wardrobe of *Peyton Place*, the television show she was filming at the time. She had the figure of a young boy and long, shiny blonde hair. She was 19; he was 49. His refusal to allow her to go to his fiftieth birthday party, because his family didn't approve, was a turning point for Farrow. The next morning she turned up late for a day of filming *Peyton Place*, and when her director complained, 'Stop this little-girl stuff! You're an actress!', she took a pair of scissors and hacked off her hair, to an inch short all over. 'No more little girl stuff,' she told the director as she handed him her hair.

The gamine crop was the making of Farrow in more ways than one. Nobody was going to tell her what to do. Sinatra did marry her, but it was on her own terms, and they divorced when she refused to turn down the starring role in *Rosemary's Baby* (1968). Farrow's hair is an expression of conviction, integrity and determination. She might look delicate and waif-like, but she is made of steel.

In *Vogue*'s August 1967 issue, under the ever-sharp eye of its editor, Diana Vreeland (see page 36),

Farrow was photographed by David Bailey in the latest Paris looks. The caption read: 'This was the year Mia Farrow … whacked off her hair, thereby raising the curtain on a new look in movie-star faces – a face with a child's brow of candour, a strong, fresh, happy eye, and pink-shell ears that point like a fawn's, behind silky little sideburns.' Farrow had marked herself out as different, a rejection of Hollywood's preference for conventional femininity, and a clear expression of rawness and honesty.

Vidal Sassoon was enlisted to perfect Farrow's crop for *Rosemary's Baby*. The haircut pays tribute to the strength of Farrow herself, who dedicated her life to her acting career, her good works (in 2000 she became a Goodwill Ambassador for UNICEF) and her brood of children (she gave birth to four and adopted ten more). Her no-nonsense spirit inspired Emma Watson to chop her hair off when she turned 20, to mark her transition from child actor to grown-up star. Michelle Williams and Halle Berry have both cropped theirs, as have Judi Dench and countless other women keen to express who they are – timeless, ageless and thoroughly of the moment.

JANE BIRKIN

UK, born 1946

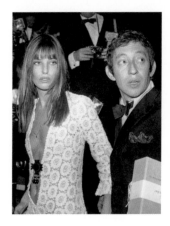

'My look is a cocktail. I'm not as nicely turned out as the French, but I don't care like the English.'

Jane Birkin's inspiration is visible everywhere, from Gucci's famous first Tom Ford collection (1994–95) to the collections for Saint Laurent by her friend Hedi Slimane. He even photographed her for Saint Laurent's advertising campaign in 2016. The editor-in-chief of *Vogue Paris*, Emmanuelle Alt, shares more than a few of Birkin's styling habits, from her long, flowing hair to her love of good jeans and a well-made man's shirt. With her lanky frame and androgynous looks, Birkin has come to personify cool French rock 'n' roll chic, an intangible quality that's more about the tilt of the head than any particular garment.

Birkin was born in London, but moved to France in the late 1960s. She brought a casual way of dressing that the Parisians weren't used to, but her look soon caught on, taking her style from futuristic Paco Rabanne shift dresses to a relaxed off-the-shoulder gypsy blouse, a glamorously cool satin blouse cut to her navel with bootleg jeans, or a delicate crochet lace dress, worn with little underneath.

Birkin's carefree, bohemian look attracted the singer Serge Gainsbourg when they met in 1968 on the film set of *Slogan*, and they became Europe's coolest, most stylish couple. That year she recorded the breathy vocals on his song 'Je t'aime … moi non plus' (originally written for Brigitte Bardot; see page 125). They lived together for 12 years and had a daughter, Charlotte, who has followed in her mother's stylish footsteps as a singer, actor and one of France's most fashionable women.

Most famously, Birkin was the inspiration for an Hermès bag. That's what happens when you sit next to the CEO of a luxury bag brand on a plane and he decides that you need a weekend bag designed especially for you. Birkin had put her signature wicker basket (she bought them for £2 in a market) in the overhead locker, and the contents fell on to the floor. She promptly drew the bag she would like, on the aeroplane sick bag. In March 2018 a Birkin sold at Christie's for £162,500, making it the most expensive bag ever sold at auction. Birkin treats hers with little reverence, of course, stuffing it with her belongings, just as she did with her famous basket.

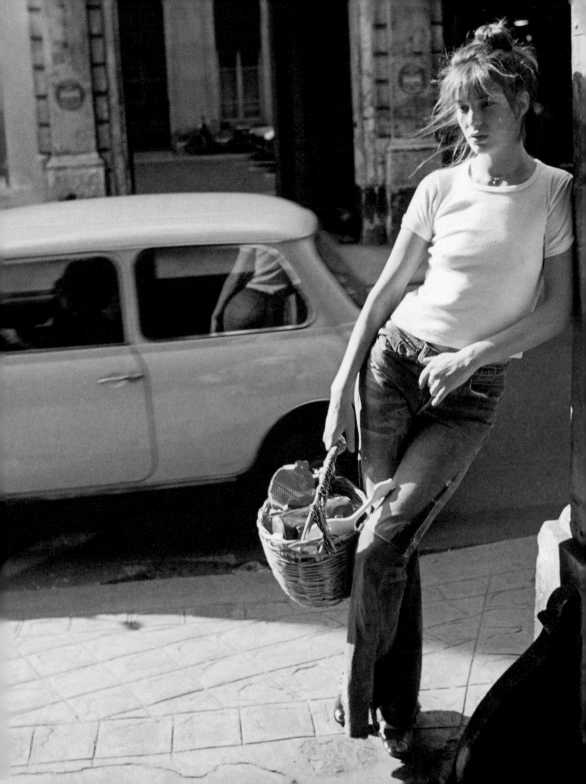

JENY HOWORTH

UK, birth date unknown

When *Elle* magazine celebrated its first birthday in November 1986, it did so with Jeny Howorth on its cover, with short blonde hair, minimal make-up and a cheeky half-smile. She was one of '*Elle*'s Belles', the girls everyone aspired to be: youthful, slightly androgynous, natural, athletic, intelligent. She led the way to a new kind of femininity. Margaret Thatcher might have been the Iron Lady in control of the country, but she didn't speak to a new generation of young women with different aspirations and values. Jeny Howorth did.

Howorth looked great in whatever she was wearing, whether strong Montana tailoring, a romantic Romeo Gigli dress, a leather jacket or a full-on Vivienne Westwood look complete with rocking-horse shoes. She could carry off very feminine clothes, making them look cool and modern, and she took masculine tailoring to another level.

The turning point for Howorth had come when she was living in New York in the early 1980s, next door to her friend the hairdresser Sam McKnight, whom she had met on her first ever shoot for the *Sunday Times*. She asked him to cut her hair, to make it easier to look after. He cropped it, and they decided to bleach it after it looked a bit patchy. The happy accident changed Howorth's life – or, at least, increased her work schedule significantly, as she hopped between shoots with Steven Meisel and Patrick Demarchelier, all keen to capture the breath of fresh air that followed her into any room.

Towards the end of the decade the young Austrian designer Helmut Lang started showing his collections of menswear and womenswear together in the same show in Paris. Howorth – who was also taking photographs for *i-D* magazine – was one of his chosen troupe, a very particular band of characters whom he used to show his industrial minimalist clothes, including Stella Tennant (see page 203) and Kirsten Owen. They walked fast and furiously around the runway, weaving their way through the audience, men and women for once equally matched. Their clothes were sometimes interchangeable. Howorth was the perfect clothes horse for this new, stark, assertive fashion.

The defining moment for Howorth was that short haircut. She wanted a hairstyle that was functional, that you would not have to wash and blow-dry every morning. She was thoroughly low-maintenance; she had things to do, places to go. And that reflected the mood of a generation of women who wanted to stride through life with the same confidence.

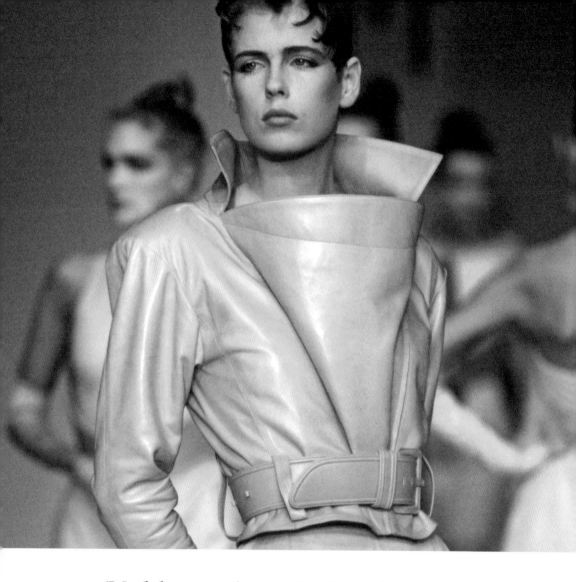

'Models were chosen for their character
and personality as much as the way they
looked. We walked as if we were walking
down the street, plus a bit of attitude.'

WINONA RYDER

USA, born 1971

'I never wanted to be any kind of role model.'

She was the pin-up girl for the 1990s, with her biker jackets and short denim skirts, slip dresses, band T-shirts and mom jeans (before mom jeans were a thing; they were just plain Levi's 501s, because that was all you could get), vintage floral dresses, bandanas as headbands, red lipstick, boys' blazers, brogues and general air of cool. She was – and, to many, still is – the coolest of the cool girls. Winona never seemed to try, but she didn't have to: she was going out with Johnny Depp.

It was as the star of the subversive teen movie *Heathers* in 1988 that Ryder rose to fame. Just 16 at the time, she was perfectly cast as Veronica, one of the mean girls who gets out of control. This dark comedy was the template for all future mean-girl films (and television shows), and has never been beaten. The colour-coded skirts and wide-shouldered double-breasted blazers the girls wore were period gems way beyond the tartan suits of *Clueless* (1995). The red scrunchie and powder-blue tights have become cult wardrobe staples for any *Heathers* fan.

Ryder's hair was as inspiring as her clothes. Her neat *Heathers* bob morphed into a choppy, shaggy cut for the Gen X film *Reality Bites* (1994). Her perfect pixie cut for *The Alien: Resurrection* in 1997 spawned endless copies.

In 2002, after being convicted of shoplifting clothes worth over $5,000 from Saks in Beverly Hills, Ryder inspired a cult T-shirt – the sort of thing she would have worn herself – with the slogan 'Free Winona Ryder'. But in her thirties she became the focus for the fashion set once more, and a muse for Marc Jacobs (who loved the irony that she had shoplifted one of his jumpers), who used her in his campaign the year after her arrest, as well as making her the face of his beauty range and his campaign in 2015. He described her as 'a brilliant mind, talent, and physical beauty like no other.'

Ryder appeared in H&M's Spring/Summer 2018 campaign, the perfect icon for a generation rediscovering 1990s fashion. 'There were certain things that were simply welcome,' she said of her youthful style. 'Like, suddenly it was "cool" to wear thrift store clothes, flannels, etc. That was great in the sense that it was something that everyone could afford … Then designers started making $500 flannel shirts and we were like, "huh?"'

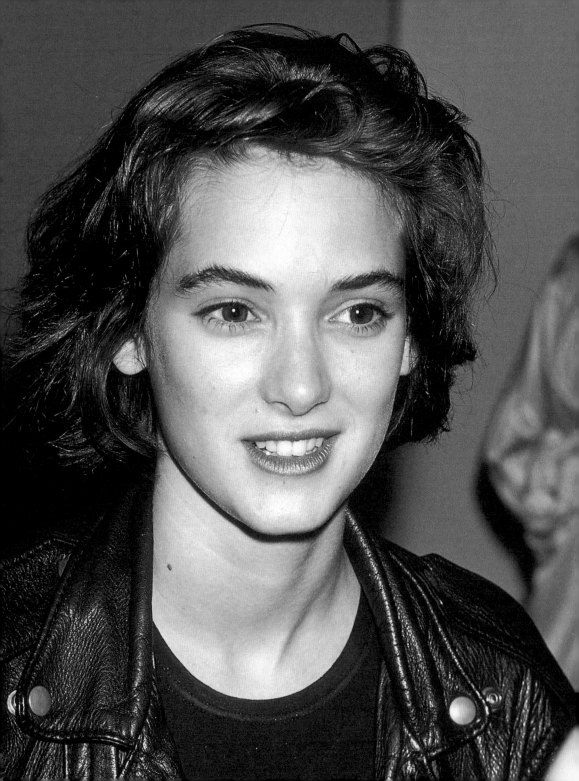

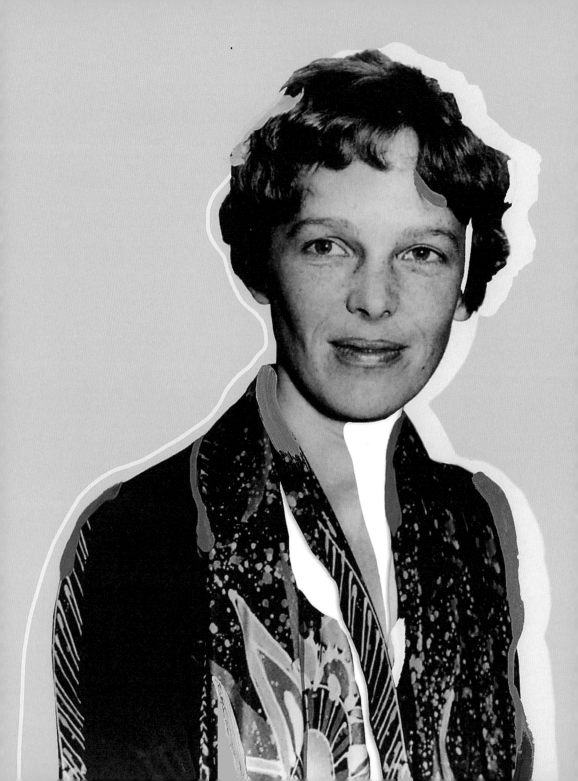

Pioneers

There are some women who are style leaders, and others who are on a mission to change the world, but there are a few who manage to do both in equal measure. These are the women who have an agenda and are determined to make their mark; how they look is simply an extension of who they are and what they do. They cannot fail to inspire us all.

AMELIA
EARHART

USA, born 1897, disappeared 1937

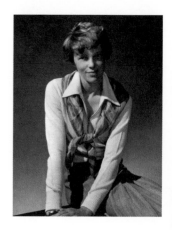

'There's more to life than being a passenger.'

Amelia Earhart, the first woman aviator to fly solo across the Atlantic, in 1932, would not have been happy about the Barbie doll made in her image to celebrate International Women's Day in March 2018. For a start, the leather jacket is far too neat and pristine. When she had her first flying lesson, in January 1921, she wore a leather flying jacket that she had slept in for three nights to make sure it looked sufficiently worn in. She wanted to be taken seriously – and of course she was. By 1937, when her plane famously disappeared over the Pacific, somewhere near Howland Island, she was a household name.

Earhart's image and clothes were a crucial part of her story and mythology. As president of the Ninety-Nines, an organization of women aviators, she designed a flight suit with women in mind, rather than the standard created for men. Hers was made as a two-piece and was advertised in *Vogue*.

In 1933 Earhart and her entrepreneurial husband, George Putnam, launched a clothing line, Amelia Earhart Fashions, as a way to fund her expeditions. It was one of the first celebrity fashion lines. Earhart told the press at the time that she had included 'something

characteristic of aviation, a parachute cord or tie or belt, a ball-bearing belt buckle, wing bolts and nuts for buttons'. The pieces were affordable, and patterns were distributed through women's magazines for home dressmaking.

The 'Queen of the Air' was effectively a lifestyle brand before that was even a thing, and her designs were sold in 50 stores, including Macy's. In 1934 Earhart, who smiled with her mouth closed to hide the gap in her teeth, was voted one of the ten best-dressed women in America. Her look was catching on with everyone from Marlene Dietrich and Katharine Hepburn in Hollywood (see pages 102 and 106) to ordinary women who were adopting this thoroughly modern wardrobe of trousers, easy-to-wash shirts and zip-up jackets.

Earhart's own rugged style – she crossed the Atlantic in a suede Abercrombie & Fitch jacket – could easily be worn by the modern (wannabe) aviator today. She has inspired countless designers, including Jean Paul Gaultier, who based his Autumn/Winter 2009–10 collection at Hermès on her, complete with bomber jackets and flight goggles.

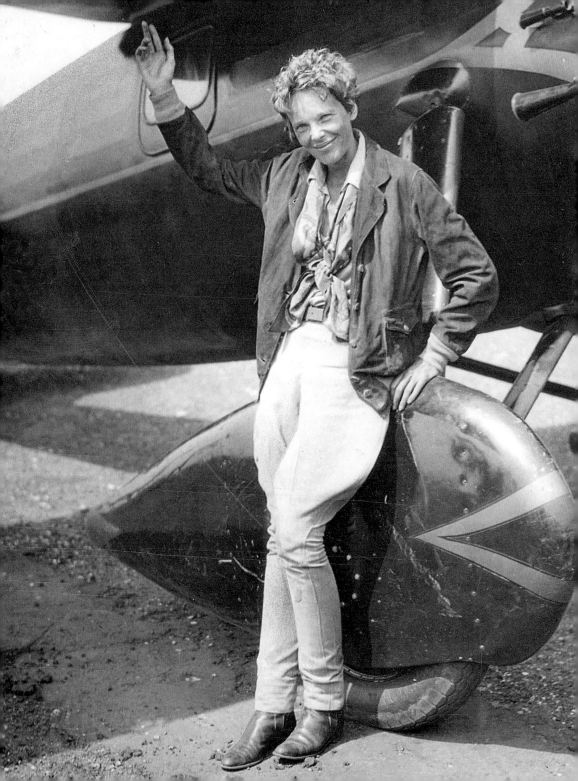

JOSEPHINE BAKER

USA, 1906–1975

'I wasn't really naked. I simply didn't have any clothes on.'

Josephine Baker was the best-loved and most highly paid performer in Jazz Age Paris. As the star turn of the Folies Bergère, she performed her *danse sauvage* nude but for a skirt of bananas, an exotic (and erotic) colonial fantasy. She may have been part of the joke, but she was laughing too (as was Beyoncé, who paid homage to her by performing in a banana skirt in 2006). Baker's act was risqué and avant-garde, in tune with the African-influenced Art Deco movement that was sweeping through Paris in 1925, the year she arrived there to perform as part of the Revue nègre.

But Baker's influence went far beyond her extraordinary routines and dazzling costumes. In the 1930s she became the first black woman to take the lead role in a feature film. Such was her influence that she marketed a skin-darkening lotion, Bakerskin, and hair oil, Bakerhair, for women desperate to 'get the look'. During World War II she served as part of the Free French resistance movement, carrying valuable intelligence for the allies and earning herself the Legion of Honour. Although she settled in France, she was a high-profile supporter of the civil rights movement in America, and the only female speaker at the March on Washington in 1963.

Baker was an inspiration to the designers – from Christian Dior to Elsa Schiaparelli (see page 81) – who dressed her, to Pablo Picasso, who drew her, to Ernest Hemingway and to Jean Cocteau, who created the banana skirt and said of her that 'eroticism has found a style.'

With her jangle of statement earrings and costume jewellery, her streamlined Marcel-waved hair (the celebrity hairdresser Antoine de Paris created her lacquered wigs, and they became all the rage) and her Jazz Age zigzags, feathers and geometric costumes, Baker was an extraordinary fusion of fashion, performance, music and activism. You need only look at her infectious smile to realize that anything is possible.

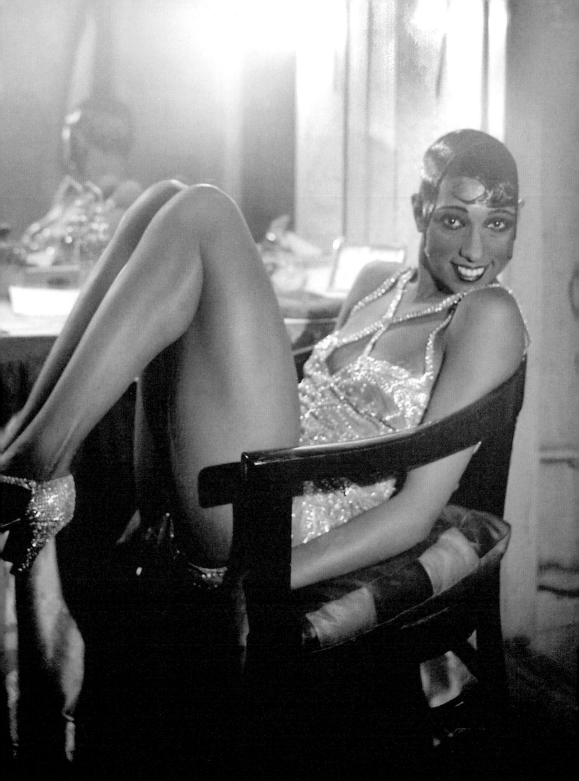

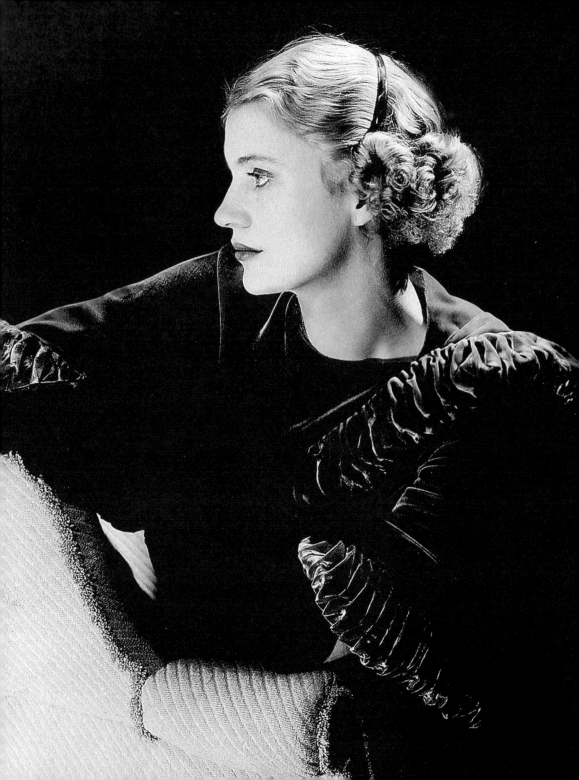

LEE MILLER

USA, 1907–1977

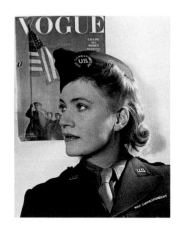

*'If I need to pee, I pee in the road;
if I have a letch for someone,
I hop into bed with him.'*

The story goes that in 1926 Condé Nast saved Lee Miller from being run over by a truck as she crossed the road in Manhattan. He was struck by her beauty, which became her passport to untold adventures and love affairs. After being introduced by Nast to the editor of *Vogue*, Edna Woolman Chase, Miller posed for the illustrator Georges Lepape. The resulting image – in which her cool blue eyes perfectly match the chic cloche hat pulled down over them – appeared on the cover of *Vogue* in March 1927. Miller became a favourite of the photographer Edward Steichen and a fixture on the fashionable party scene. Her daringly bobbed hair, boyish figure and flapper style embodied *Vogue*'s new reflection of a modern age.

Steichen introduced Miller to the work of the photographer Man Ray, whom she tracked down in Paris, informing him that she was going to be his student. They embarked on a three-year affair, during which she accidentally discovered the solarization technique for which he became famous. Miller's lack of inhibition enabled her to bring her surrealist eye to everything she photographed, from a fashion-accessory still life to the front line, a place where women photographers were not supposed to venture.

When Miller signed up as an army war correspondent, she bought her uniform from Savile Row, and she proved a daring and unflinching chronicler of the conflict, becoming the first photographer (along with her comrade David Scherman) to document the atrocities of Dachau, as well as directing her lens towards how women were coping on the home front. She famously stamped the mud of Dachau into Hitler's bathmat before being photographed (by Scherman) in the bath of his private apartment in Munich at the end of the war.

Miller changed the way we look at war, photographing gypsy women and brothel workers from the camp, and homeless children, as well as the violence of the battlefield. Such images would haunt her for the rest of her life.

BILLIE HOLIDAY

USA, 1915–1959

Nicknamed 'Lady Day' by the saxophonist Lester Young (she called him 'Prez'), Billie Holiday was a fighter, not because she wanted to be, but because she had no option. The subject matter of her songs – 'Good Morning Heartache', 'I'm a Fool to Want You', 'Gloomy Sunday' – spoke of exploitative relationships and emotional turmoil as well as civil-rights abuses, giving a pretty accurate picture of her short and tragic life. She did not shy away from speaking out. In 1939 she recorded the song 'Strange Fruit', which protested against the lynching of African Americans, and which she would perform throughout her career.

For most of her public life, however, Holiday's star shone bright in satin and sparkling jewels, and she thrilled and chilled her audiences as they listened to her in smoky underground nightclubs such as the Downbeat and the Alhambra in New York. She had pulled herself out of poverty by singing in clubs, and was scouted and signed to Brunswick Records in 1935. In the 1930s she sang with Artie Shaw's orchestra, one of the first black women to sing with a white band. As the highest-paid singer on the jazz-club circuit, she was earning almost $1,000 a week, allowing her to indulge her love of fashion with fine jewels, fancy gowns and fur coats. She had a great sense of style and amazing grace, and provided the shot of glamour that any jazz band needed in her lavish floral gowns, satin cocktail dresses and strappy platform shoes. She had to live up to her aristocratic nickname, after all.

Holiday's look (and sound) has been referenced by numerous women since, including Sade (see page 210), Amy Winehouse (see page 181) and Erykah Badu. There is something deeply romantic and nostalgic about Holiday, particularly the exotic flowers she wore in her hair. It is said that she adopted them originally to hide a patch of hair that she had burned with a curling iron, but they quickly became her trademark; she must have loved the romance and drama they brought to her look, and their fragrance, as delicate and intangible as her voice.

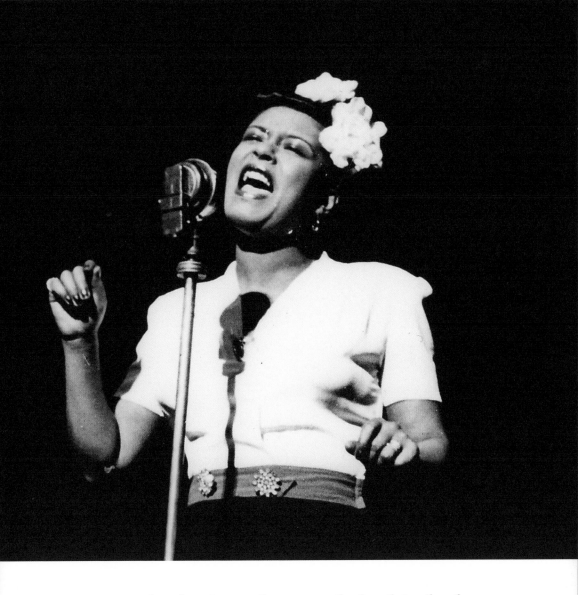

'People don't understand the kind of
fight it takes to record what you want to
record the way you want to record it.'

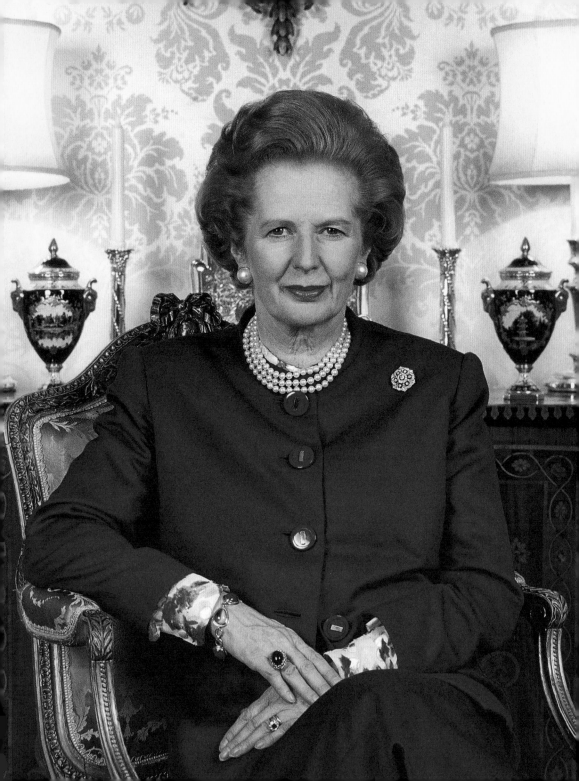

MARGARET THATCHER

UK, 1925–2013

'If you do not wear a brooch or pearls, the outfit is not quite finished.'

Margaret Thatcher polarizes opinion, when it comes to both her politics and her dress sense. When in 2015 the Victoria and Albert Museum in London was offered some of her iconic suits for its twentieth-century dress collection, it declined politely, saying the clothes were not of good enough quality to be in the museum. What a put-down for a woman who prided herself on making the most of herself and understood, more than most, the symbolism and power of a smart blue skirt suit! She favoured buttons like knuckledusters, a weighty, no-nonsense handbag (which she used as a metaphorical weapon against anyone who dared to oppose her), a solid helmet of hair and a silky pussy bow at the neck.

Thatcher was a pioneer. When she was first elected a Member of Parliament, in 1959, she was just one of 25 women among 650 men. The attitude towards women in UK politics at the time was at best patronizing and at worst downright misogynistic. For her to become leader of the Conservative party, and in 1979 the first female British prime minister, was not so much breaking the glass ceiling as firing a rocket through it and going to the moon and back again. Indeed, her clothes were the equivalent of a space suit or a form of armour, taking her into uncharted territory.

In 1990 Thatcher talked about how she chose her clothes: 'I much prefer something tailored, it suits me, I can put it on and forget it and I like the recipe of a jacket and skirt and it looks tailored, it looks executive. But also in a strange way, you know, a very tailored thing with a special neckline can also look very soft.' She thought anything that deviated from her uniform distracted from what she was saying, and her plain power suit became the mode of dressing for any woman who wanted to be taken seriously, whether in the boardroom or on the soapbox. Its influence lives on in the wardrobes of the world's prominent female politicians today: Theresa May, Angela Merkel and Hillary Clinton all owe a boxy-shouldered jacket or two to the Iron Lady.

GLORIA STEINEM

USA, born 1934

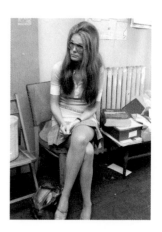

As a young journalist in the 1960s, Gloria Steinem faced constant sexism and was derided for trading on her looks, as if being beautiful made her a less serious person. But there was no word for sexual harassment back then; 'It was just called "life",' she said. She liked clothes – shock horror, a feminist who had manicures, spent time at the hairdresser and wore heels! – but she did not see why she should be defined by the way she looked.

Steinem had become something of a celebrity after writing a two-part story for *Show Magazine* in 1963, exposing the reality of life as a Playboy Bunny. After the piece was published, Hugh Hefner stopped the practice of requiring the Bunnies to have gynaecological examinations as part of the job application process, but Steinem was stigmatized and not taken seriously because she had herself gone undercover – as a Playboy Bunny.

In 1968 Steinem was invited to join the staff writers of a new magazine, *New York*. One of the many subjects she tackled was abortion rights. She was among the one in three American women who

had needed an abortion, and who didn't have a safe place to talk about it. Her story became one of the first mainstream reports on the burgeoning women's movement, but it wasn't enough. She realized that, even as a reporter covering political campaigns, she was seen as the 'pretty girl' in the office. 'I was doing politics, but even at the magazine I was still the girl writer,' she said, 'and the guys there, whom I loved, their advice about feminism was, "Don't get involved with those crazy women." I thought, These guys are my friends, and they don't know who I am, because I haven't said.' Her magazine, *Ms.*, was as loud a statement as she could make. Launched in 1972, it became the platform for a generation of women to read about previously unreported topics that were important to them – and it was written and controlled by women.

Steinem hasn't stopped since: at the Women's March in Washington, DC, in 2017, she took the stand alongside her sisters-in-arms with a speech that was more powerful and more necessary than ever. The battle lines are changing, but the fight goes on.

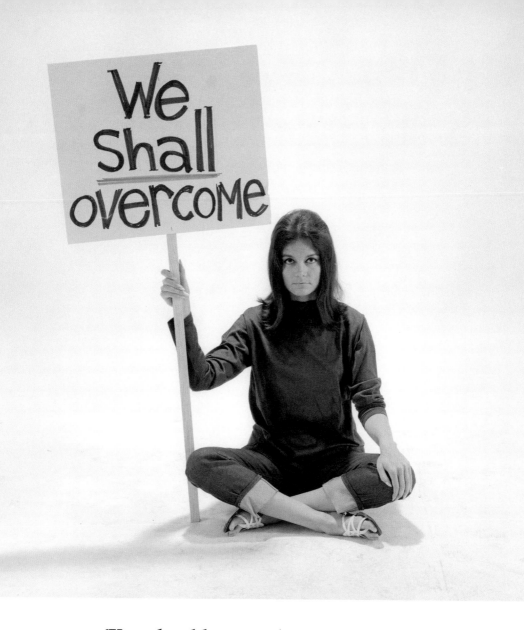

'You should write about take-no-
shit women like me. Girls need to
know they can break the rules.'

KATHARINE HAMNETT

UK, born 1947

'I'd always believed the trick was to be successful and be a decent human being as well.'

As is often the way with pioneers, the designer Katharine Hamnett has been ahead of her time with many things, not just boiler suits, sportswear and a flagship store that made a star of its architect, Nigel Coates, long before Prada put architects in the fashion limelight. She's changed the way we look at – and how we think about – everything from pesticides in cotton to nuclear arms, war, Brexit and acid rain. If Hamnett had her way, we would have somehow saved the sea, the bees, the NHS, for heaven's sake – *and* controlled climate change. In short, the future would be in much better shape.

In 1987, when she wore her 58% Don't Want Pershing T-shirt under a raincoat to a drinks party at 10 Downing Street, Hamnett was letting her clothes speak for her – just a few words that couldn't be missed. Even before the days of instant social-media coverage, this became a very famous image, a direct way of speaking truth to power.

Thanks to Hamnett's lead, we now put slogans on our T-shirts at the drop of a pink pussy hat. She was using fashion as a vehicle for positive change before anyone even thought about sewing their political beliefs in sequins. For Hamnett, along with the millions of women and men she has inspired and galvanized into action, getting dressed in the morning is a political act.

Two years after her Downing Street protest, Hamnett learned about the way cotton is produced and the detrimental effect it was having on the environment as well as on tens of thousands of cotton farmers in India and Africa. She went on a mission to change the industry, asking her suppliers for organic cotton. At the time, she was almost a lone voice. But 30 years later sustainability is a huge buzzword, and the industry cannot grow enough organic cotton to keep up with demand.

Hamnett recently relaunched her 1980s classics, and she remains a tireless campaigner across a range of topics. Sales of her Choose Love T-shirt have raised thousands for the charity Help Refugees, and, of course, it's made from 100 per cent organic cotton. Ultimately, she has shown how fashion can be used to question the status quo and make positive change.

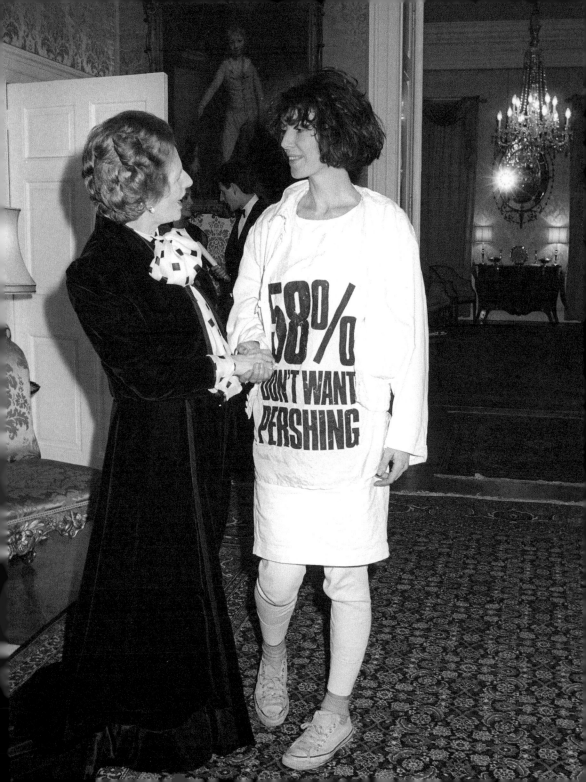

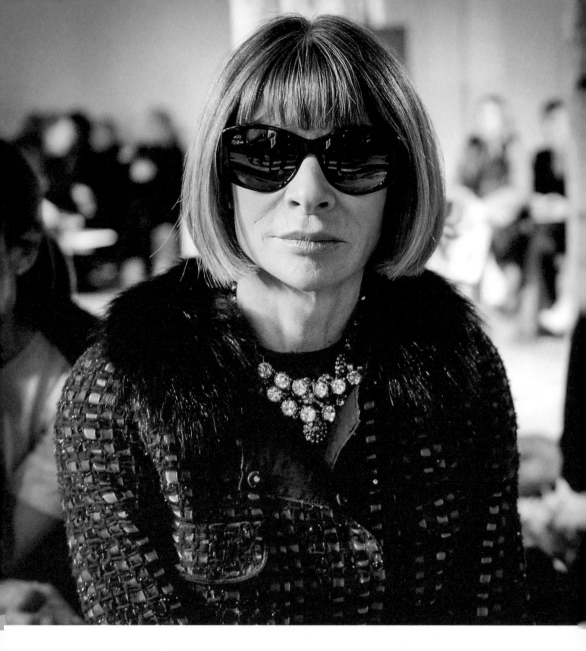

'If my style is too direct for some,
maybe they should toughen up a bit.'

ANNA WINTOUR

UK, born 1949

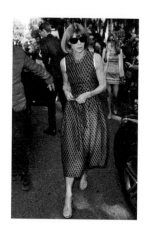

The razor-sharp bob, the inscrutable dark glasses, the immaculate Chanel suit cut to the knee, the bare legs, the elegant Manolo Blahnik slingback heels: Anna Wintour spells power, and for 30 years her word has been fashion gospel. When she became the editor of American *Vogue* in 1988, her first cover starred the model Michaela Bercu wearing a Christian Lacroix jewelled jacket with a pair of stonewashed jeans. It shook up the industry, signalling a new direction after a decade of big hair and armour-plated shoulders.

While Wintour's own style never wavers – never seen in head-to-toe black, she favours lighter, often iridescent colours, preferably by Chanel, with two or three strings of her favourite crystal necklaces – her *Vogue* is a champion of the new. 'Fashion is not about looking back. It's always about looking forward,' she has said, and she has made it her business to nurture the hottest new talent.

Whatever Wintour does, she does with absolute conviction, whether it be her endorsement of Hillary Clinton as president (and her subsequent needling of Donald Trump) or her commitment to raising funds for the Metropolitan Museum with the annual star-studded glamour-fest that is the Met Ball.

Wintour was born in London, left school at 18 and went to work as a junior fashion editor at *Harper's Bazaar* in New York in 1975, in her mid-twenties. In 1981 she was made fashion editor at *New York* magazine. Her work caught the eye of Alexander Liberman, the legendary editorial director of American *Vogue*, who offered her a job as the magazine's creative director. When she returned to London in 1986 to edit British *Vogue* for two years, she earned herself the nickname 'Nuclear Wintour'. She was, of course, the inspiration for Miranda Priestly, the icy, tunnel-visioned editor-in-chief in *The Devil Wears Prada* (2003). In 2009 the documentary film *The September Issue* followed Wintour in real life as she prepared for the most important issue of the year, making her a mainstream celebrity.

Wintour's *Vogue* continues to reflect changes in fashion and society, most memorably including Kim Kardashian and Kanye West shot by Annie Leibovitz for the April 2014 issue. The shoot signifies the power and popularity of this first couple of social media – and Wintour's brilliance at taking the pulse of society and channelling it into her magazine.

STELLA McCARTNEY

UK, born 1971

'Everyone can do simple things to make a difference, and every little bit really does count.'

When Stella McCartney launched her first collection under her own name, in partnership with the Gucci group (later to become Kering) in 2001, it seemed unthinkable that her ethos of no animal cruelty – plastic shoes! fake fur! non-leather jackets! – would fit at the heart of Italy's luxury-goods industry, built as it is on a love affair with animal skin. So Gucci's announcement in 2017 that it was stopping using fur because it 'just wasn't modern' was proof that to make change, you must be part of the machine.

McCartney's animal-rights activism stems from her belief as a lifelong vegetarian that it is wrong to kill animals for meat. Her mother, Linda McCartney, was a phenomenal influence, not just on her vegetarianism but also on her fashion aesthetic, from her love of blazers, ruffled blouses, culottes, A-line skirts and dressing-gown wrap coats to the masculine edges and vaguely 1970s bohemian look that typify her style. Her mother's wardrobe staples were key to her success at her first job when, fresh out of college, she took over

from Karl Lagerfeld (no less) as the creative director at Chloé.

McCartney, who in March 2018 bought back the 50 per cent of her company owned by Kering to become totally independent, has also been leading the charge for a more sustainable fashion industry. She recently teamed up with the round-the-world yachtswoman Ellen MacArthur on her mission to create a circular fashion economy, recovering waste and virgin materials from the production cycle so that in the future we will not strip the Earth of its precious resources.

McCartney has been brilliant – and unrelenting – at bringing her influential friends with her on this journey. At her degree show at Central Saint Martins in 1995 her friends Kate Moss and Naomi Campbell (see pages 22 and 21) wore her clothes on the student catwalk. These days Gwyneth Paltrow and Meghan Markle (see page 204) are proud to be part of Team Stella. McCartney tells us it's the small things that make a difference – such as washing clothes at 30°C – and I for one am happy to take her lead.

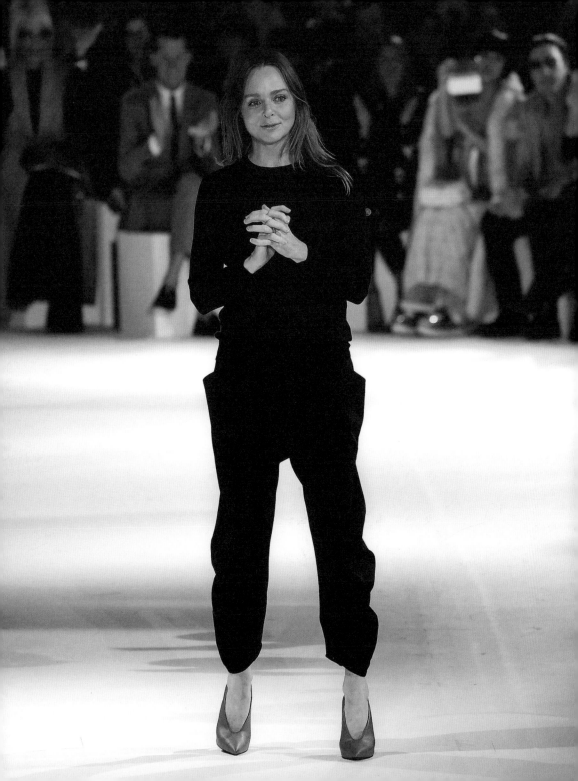

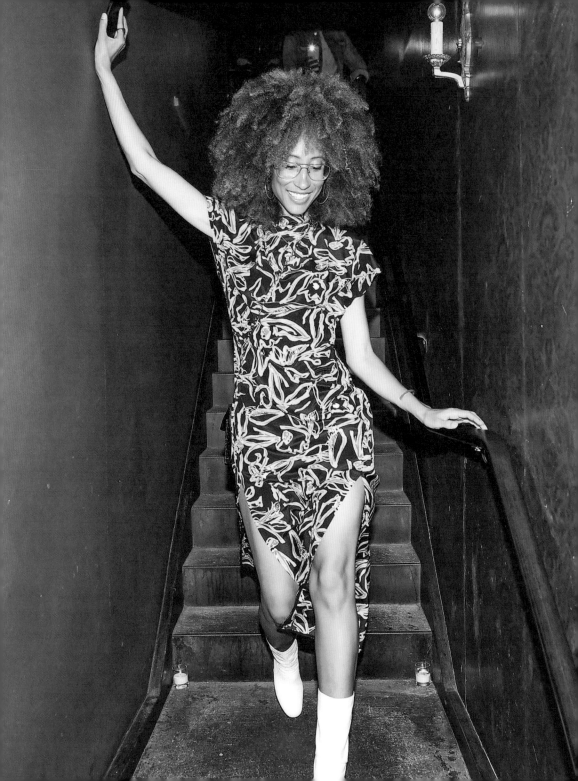

ELAINE WELTEROTH

USA, born 1987

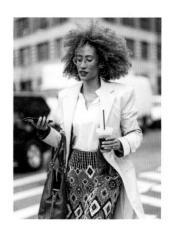

'Activism is being authentically who you are in public.'

With her curly 'fro, her geeky specs, her penchant for berets made in Ethiopia by her ethical fashion friend Aurora James, her trademark white boots and her natural affinity with Alessandro Michele's Gucci, Elaine Welteroth could not be a better spokeswoman for Generation Woke. She came to prominence not because she was the youngest Condé Nast editor, or the second African-American woman to become editor of a Condé Nast title, but because she gave *Teen Vogue* a political voice at a time when a newly politically engaged generation really needed one. She became editor of the title in May 2016 at the age of 29, having previously joined the magazine as beauty editor. Welteroth's approach is direct, upbeat, positive and so full of life and opinion that you can't help but be swept along with her.

With Welteroth as beauty director (Condé Nast's first ever black beauty director) and then editor, *Teen Vogue* became a hotbed of youthful political activism in the face of the Trump presidency, a publication that young (and some older) people felt was speaking good sense, and, most importantly, the truth. Politics, fashion and culture have become mixed and writers are encouraged to talk authentically about subjects such as cultural appreciation as opposed to cultural appropriation.

Welteroth is the figurehead for a newly inclusive, highly conscious, gender-fluid fashion and media industry. She helps to create a more level playing field, where underdogs, outcasts and people who have previously not felt included in the conversation can take centre stage. She doesn't just write about this stuff, she lives it. She loves clothes, make-up and skincare, but she brings a cultural, political and feminist perspective to everything she does. She's big on collaboration and an endless fount of big-sisterly advice, in many ways continuing the work started by Gloria Steinem (see page 154) in the 1960s.

Welteroth left *Teen Vogue* in 2018 and signed with the talent agency CAA. After a cameo role in the ABC comedy *Black-ish*, she has taken on a writing role on *Grown-ish*. She uses Instagram as her discussion pad, engaging with her followers – 292,000 of them, and rising.

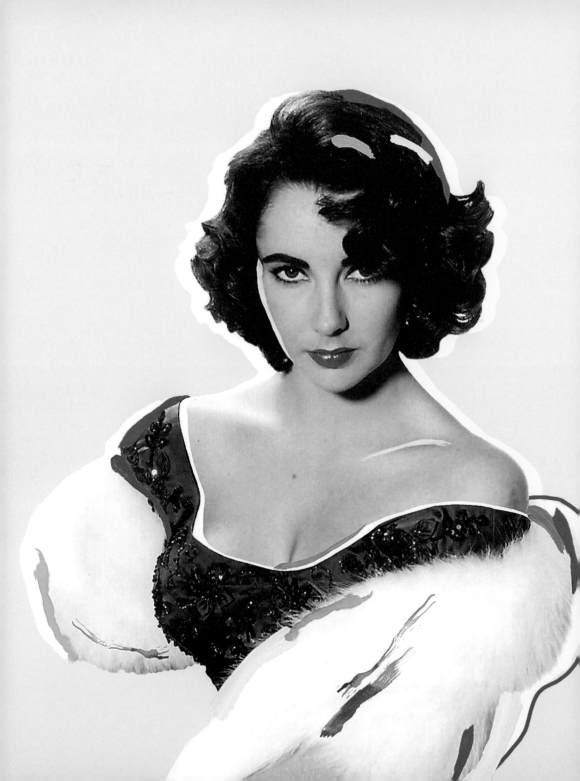

Cleopatras

Eyebrows as magnificent as the temples built in her honour, eyelids painted shimmering malachite green, jet-black hair (lots of it) and ears heavy with gold: that is how we imagine Cleopatra VII, the last great ruler of Egypt. But in fact, her spirit and her fiery, unstoppable energy live on. For some, the influence is merely a stylistic one – the strong line of kohl that says: 'Look into my eyes, don't mess with me.' These women are a force of nature. Yes, they say, you have the power to create your own mythology. Just let anyone try to stop you!

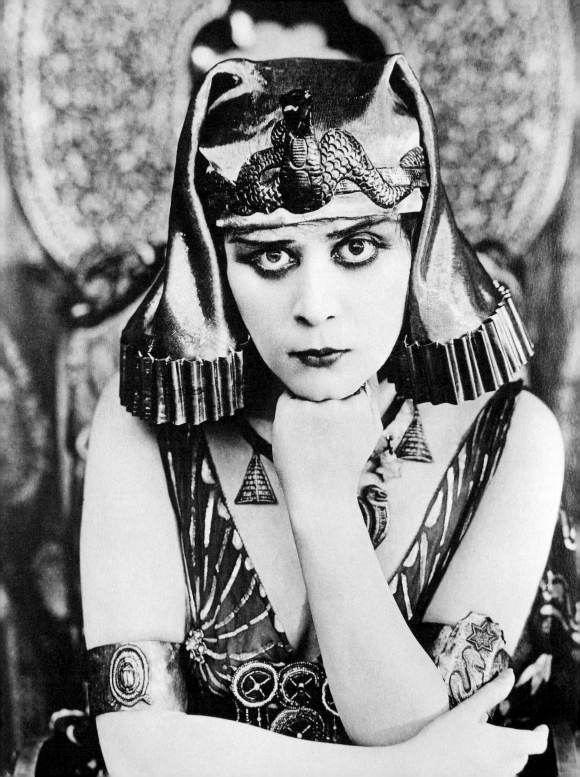

THEDA BARA

USA, 1885–1955

'To be good is to be forgotten. I'm going to be so bad I'll always be remembered.'

Theda Bara took her surname from her Swiss grandfather, Francis Bara de Coppet, changing it from the less romantic-sounding Goodman in 1917. By then she was already a famous screen actress, the original sex symbol.

Bara appeared in almost 20 films, but tragically most of them – all silent – have been lost or were destroyed in a fire at Fox's archive. She was one of the first creations of the movie PR machine. Although she had Swiss-Polish parentage (she was born in Cincinnati to a tailor and a housewife), she was publicized as having been born in the shadow of the Sphinx, the offspring of a French actress and an Italian artist, who spent her childhood playing on the Pyramids and learning the ways of the serpent. Her hair was dyed black to emphasize her exotic looks.

And it worked. Bara was the original wanton woman, the ultimate vamp. For women, she was mesmerizing, the personification of unfettered sexuality in a world where women were newly liberated from their corsets, and awakening to the possibilities for spreading their wings. For men, she was altogether more disturbing, an otherworldly creature who threatened to put them under her spell and have her wicked way with them. They might have been tempted – can

you blame them? – but they feared for their lives.

For the stars of silent movies, it was all about expression. Clara Bow had the lips; Louise Brooks the geometric features to match her bob. But Bara's expressive features, emphasized with crude kohl and dark shadows for the cameras, were altogether unsettling. Her influence was as much about a state of mind as about a look. She was not soft and compliant; rather, seemingly untameable, she looked as though she was ready to suck your blood at any opportunity. She took her roles seriously, although she was usually cast as the vamp or the femme fatale in such films as *Cleopatra* (1917), *Salomé* and *The She-Devil* (both 1918). To research her role as Cleopatra, she spent months with the director of Egyptology at the Metropolitan Museum of Art in New York. Sadly, only a few stills survive from the film.

Bara was mystical, and believed in the occult. In many ways, she has more in common with the Pre-Raphaelite paintings of mythical creatures such as John William Waterhouse's *Lady of Shalott* (1888) or Dante Gabriel Rossetti's *Pandora* (1871) than the thoroughly modern, emancipated women of the Jazz Age who were to take her place on the silver screen.

ELIZABETH TAYLOR

UK, 1932–2011

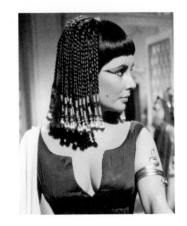

'There are many doors to be opened and I'm not afraid to look behind them.'

Elizabeth Taylor was perfectly cast as Cleopatra in the film of 1963. The story of Taylor and her co-star Richard Burton was almost as dramatic as that of Antony and Cleopatra. Certainly, as the highest-paid actress in Hollywood at the time – $1 million for the film that nearly bankrupted the studio – she was almost as rich and powerful as the Egyptian ruler herself. Burton fell under her spell: the couple were to divorce and marry twice, and the jewels he gave her were the stuff of legend. The 33-carat diamond ring from Harry Winston; La Peregrina, the pearl that was discovered in the sixteenth century and became part of the Crown Jewels of Spain; and the seventeenth-century heart-shaped diamond that was the inspiration for the Taj Mahal were equal to anything Cleopatra herself might have owned.

Taylor would not have had it any other way. She did what she wanted, as she wanted, with whoever she wanted. She was ruled by her heart and her instinct in everything she did. When the head of RKO Pictures, Howard Hughes, tried to arrange a marriage with her in return for $1 million, she apparently laughed and chose her own husband, Conrad 'Nicky' Hilton, the wealthy son of the hotel magnate, in 1950. She was just 18 and divorced him the following year.

Taylor had a similarly voracious – if less fickle – appetite for fashion. The fashion world loved her, not least because when she liked something she would buy it in multiples of ten or twenty. Women – and men – lusted after her perfect nose, violet eyes, thick eyebrows and ample cleavage. As a Hollywood star, she became an incredible source of inspiration, whether it was the Grecian draped white dress she wore as Maggie the Cat in *Cat on a Hot Tin Roof* (1958; it's still a wardrobe staple today – look no further than Lupita Nyong'o's Oscars dress in 2015; see page 118), the slip she wore for her Oscar-winning role in *Butterfield 8* (1960) or the angular eyebrows and exaggerated eyeliner for her role as Cleopatra.

Taylor reinvented herself many times, with bouffants and puffballs, caftans and Versace prints. When she died in 2011, she left over 1,000 pieces of clothing and more than 200 handbags, including pieces by Pucci, Versace, Valentino, Dior and John Galliano. She lived life to the full, generously, stylishly, passionately, sometimes sensationally, but always on her own terms.

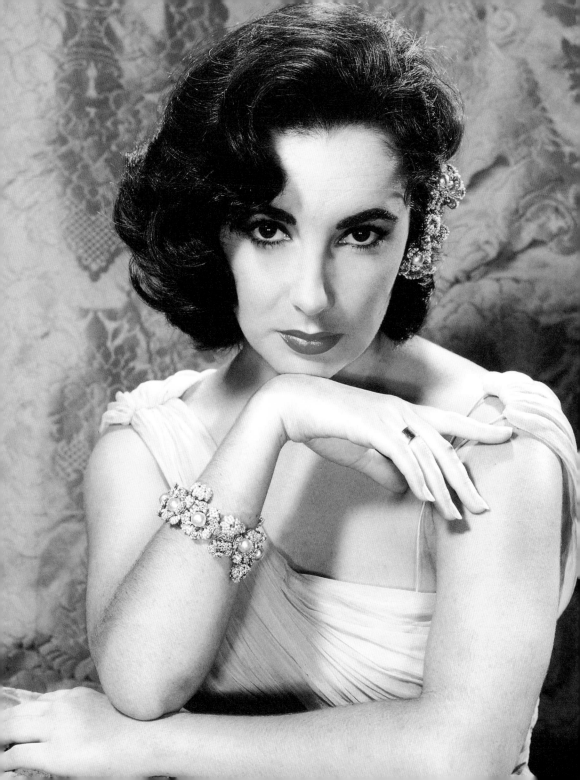

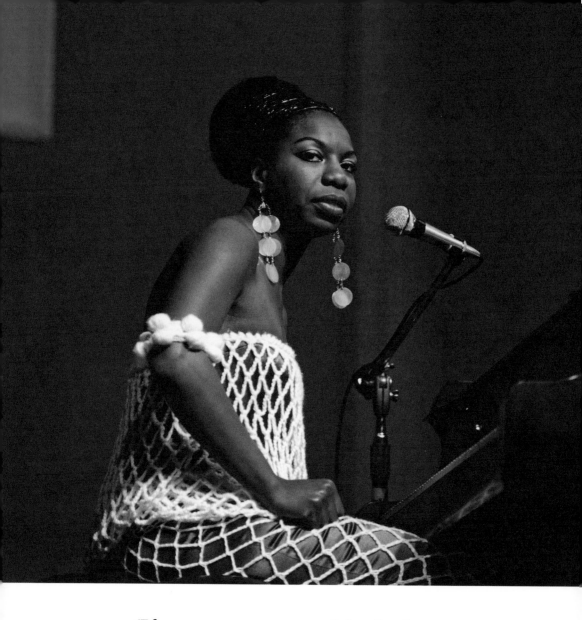

*'If you come out and look the way
you want to look, you will create a
mood before you open your mouth!'*

NINA SIMONE

USA, 1933–2003

She was fierce. She was angry. She was proud. Nina Simone's voice and music have seared themselves into the consciousness of generations, from her hits 'Feeling Good' (1965) and 'My Baby Just Cares for Me' (1958) to the civil rights anthem 'To Be Young, Gifted and Black' (1969).

Born into a middle-class family, Eunice Waymon created the persona of Nina Simone when she took a job in a piano bar in Atlantic City in 1954, in order to hide what she was doing from her mother. It was a way of earning money, but far less respectable than her classical music education at the Juilliard School in New York City. As Simone, however, she was free to express herself as she wanted, to write songs about disenfranchisement, inequality, racism, sexism and anger at the injustice of society.

The blackness of Simone's skin is what powered her, what shaped her experience of the world and the way the world treated her. She once commented that she was never on the cover of a magazine such as *Ebony* and *Jet* because they wanted 'white-looking' women, such as Diana Ross. With her strong, African features, she did not look like other women of colour who were given a platform on stage or screen. Her physique, sitting upright at the piano, totally in control of her keyboard, her clear, accusatory eyes lined with kohl, her muscular shoulders bare, a piece of statement jewellery around her neck, gave her a regal appearance that demanded absolute respect.

Simone was fearless in her performances and often disdainful of her white audiences, who, no matter how sympathetic they were to her cause, could never truly understand what it was to be her. She became the voice of the civil rights movement, and her extraordinary, gut-wrenching performance of the song 'Brown Baby' (1962), an anthem of her times, was every bit as powerful (although darker and more pessimistic) as Martin Luther King's 'I Have a Dream' speech.

She was often accused of being stroppy and difficult, a bit of a prima donna, but in fact Simone suffered from problems with her mental health, possibly a form of bipolar disorder. She also endured a dysfunctional relationship with her controlling husband and manager, Andrew Stroud. But she gave a voice and a sense of power and pride to millions of women who felt shunned by society. 'Birds flying high, you know how I feel,' she sang. She made them feel free – in their hearts, at least.

RONNIE SPECTOR

USA, born 1943

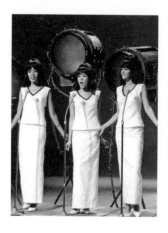

'We had the skirts with the slits up the side, sort of tough, sort of Spanish Harlem cool, but sweet too.'

Ronnie Spector grew up in Spanish Harlem, New York City, a beautiful mix of African American, Cherokee and Irish American. Her older sister Estelle was sent for singing lessons (the family couldn't afford to send Ronnie too) and, with their cousin Nedra, the pair would perform for family functions. The trio started to perform as the Ronettes in the early 1960s.

It was Ronnie's emotional vocals that meant they were played on the radio, but it was the girls' style that got them noticed on stage, not least when they performed on tour with the Rolling Stones and the Beatles between 1964 and 1966. They unleashed a raw, edgy sexuality that was mixed with sweetness and innocence at a time when teenagers were finding new ways of expressing who they were, how they looked and what they were feeling. 'We had attitude. When

the three Ronettes walked onstage, people went nuts because we were different,' Spector told the *Guardian* in 2014. 'We wore tight dresses when everyone else wore flared dresses, we had long hair when people had short hair; it was like the Beatles and the Stones wearing suits – it made them different.'

Madonna (see page 51) once said she wanted to look the way the Ronettes sounded, but their style has influenced a whole host of women since, not least Amy Winehouse (see page 181): the eyeliner flick, the beehive with a fringe and a ponytail, the coquettish girl-next-door mixed with a don't-mess-with-me rock 'n' roll edge – the original bad girls of rock. 'We had girls who wanted to wear their hair like us, in beehives, the Chinese bangs, the long braid!' says Ronnie, who continues to perform and still backcombs her hair.

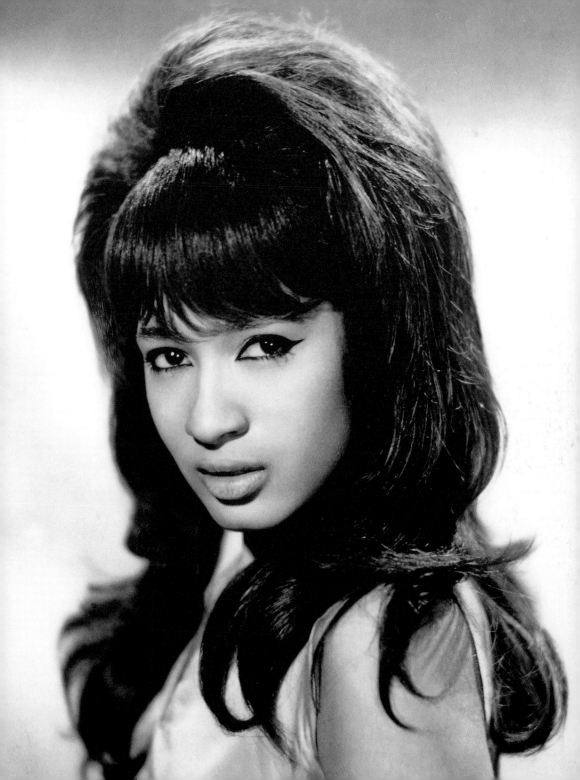

SIOUXSIE SIOUX

UK, born 1957

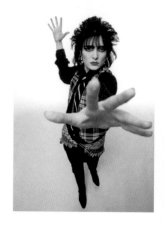

'There is a fun, flippant side to me, of course. But I would much rather be known as the Ice Queen.'

It's difficult not to be spellbound by the hypnotic, relentless music of Siouxsie and the Banshees, and by Siouxsie herself – her punky black hair; her pale, unearthly complexion; her pointy Clara Bow lips; her crudely drawn eyebrows. She snarled, she was abrasive, she was mysterious, wild and unpredictable. She was a powerful communicator, a true Cleopatra in that she was at one with her sexuality and her ability to reign supreme in a man's world. In Irish mythology, banshees were old hags dressed in dark shrouds, who would shriek and scream when someone died. Sioux was thrillingly dark. No wonder all her fans wanted to paint their bedrooms black.

'Snapped, harsh, asexual, she wears shorts/short skirts for freedom of movement,' wrote Paul Morley in the *New Musical Express* in 1978. 'Her make-up, which eerily transforms her nervous, wistful, pale face into the hard-lined clown-tragedian, is the one concession to the audience.' Sioux's look was a powerful mix of fetish, dominatrix, vamp, anarchist, mystic, witch, 1920s silent-movie femme fatale – a Theda Bara (see page 167) for the 1970s and 1980s. In their brilliant book *Women & Fashion* (1989), Caroline Evans and Minna Thornton describe Sioux wearing a Vivienne Westwood Sex T-shirt with a photograph of a pair of women's breasts on it: 'The clothes had to be worn with both aggression and irony.'

In 1976, when Malcolm McLaren was looking for bands to perform alongside the Sex Pistols at a festival he was organizing at the 100 Club in London, Sioux said she would do it. She'd never performed before. Her first live billing was as 'Suzie' and the Banshees; the mysterious 'x' came later. She says she wanted to come across as all-powerful, and to 'make it painful for people'. True to form, she wore a buzz cut, diamanté earrings and a man's tailored jacket.

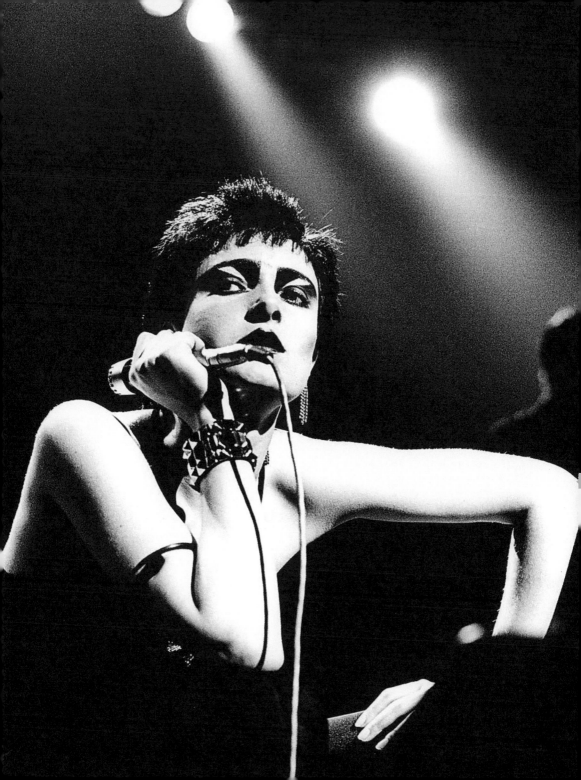

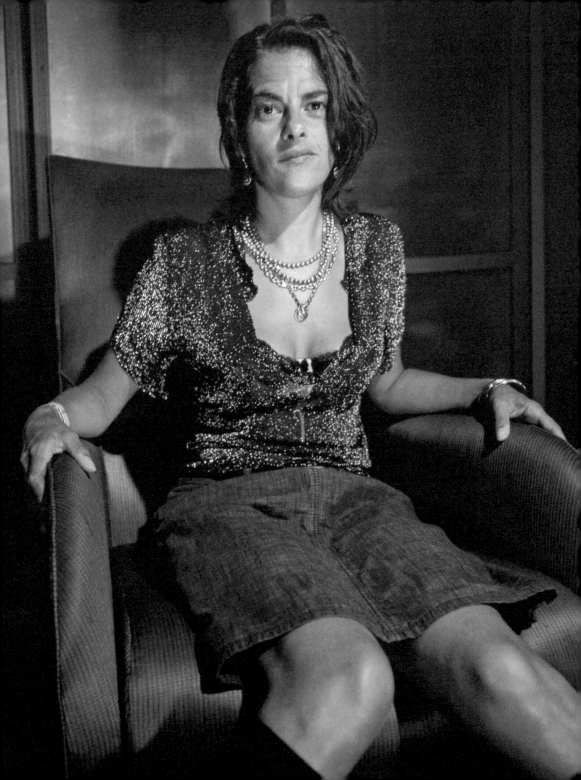

TRACEY EMIN

UK, born 1963

'I never grew up.'

The art world's rabble-rouser, Tracey Emin has never cared what people think of her. Her art is her autobiography, hers to make, and her own story to tell. 'I use myself as a subject,' she says. 'This has been a long tradition in art. Often to see the whole picture you have to start with what you know.'

Emin often uses crafts and 'women's work' to make her art, including stitching, appliqué and patchwork, in a feminist act that integrates everyday domestic life with a commentary on the reality of her sexual and emotional life. Her often crude subjects are left raw and unvarnished. She is what she is; take her or leave her. She has nothing to hide.

Emin is one of the notorious Young British Artists (with Sarah Lucas, Damien Hirst and Gary Hume, among others) who started showing together in 1988. One of her most autobiographical works, *Everyone I Have Ever Slept With 1963–1995* (1995), took the form of a tent with the names of all her lovers, friends and family appliquéd on to the inside. Perhaps her most famous work is *My Bed* (1998), shortlisted for the Turner Prize in 1999, a re-creation of her bed from when she had an emotional breakdown after a destructive relationship. She spent four days in bed in an alcoholic stupor, and was shocked when she saw the mess she had created.

Although Emin is partial to working naked in her studio, Andreas Kronthaler, the creative director of Vivienne Westwood (and the designer's husband) has described her as 'the first glamorous female artist'. Her day-to-day outfits are usually simple – men's shirts, clothes that are easy to move and work in – but her go-to designer for events is Westwood (see page 60). Emin is a great ambassador for the brand, with her unselfconscious approach and a sense that she is constantly overflowing from her clothes. There's always a bra on show, a button undone, a sense that the clothes can't quite contain the woman within.

PAT McGRATH

UK, born 1966

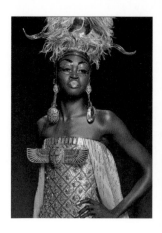

Nobody understands the power of make-up quite like Pat McGrath, the make-up artist whose extraordinary creative vision has launched hundreds of magazine covers. And nobody could upstage Cleopatra herself quite the way McGrath did with her make-up for Dior's Spring/Summer 2004 Haute Couture collection (shown above), an ancient Egyptian fantasy complete with disco death masks, gold-encrusted eyelashes and heavy lapis lazuli eyelids.

British *Vogue* has called McGrath, who was given the Isabella Blow Award for Fashion Creator by the British Fashion Council in 2017, 'the most influential makeup artist in the world'. She is known as 'Mother', and when it comes to make-up, Mother definitely knows best. She has created some of the most memorable beauty looks both in print and on the catwalk. Naomi Campbell (see page 21) says it's all about how McGrath lets the model's skin shine through. And it's true, she does make skin glow naturally. She prefers to use her fingers rather than conventional brushes and sponges, and works in a very spontaneous way.

McGrath was born in Northampton, and her introduction to the world of fashion was through her mother, Jean, a vintage-clothing hunter and self-taught dressmaker. Jean practised her talents on her daughter and taught her how to mix make-up colours for black skin, since there was little on the market at the time.

As a teenager in the 1980s McGrath became a New Romantic, slipping off to London at weekends to follow the club kids she had seen in the pages of *i-D* and *Blitz* magazines. Her big break came when she was invited on tour to Japan with Caron Wheeler, the singer with Soul II Soul. McGrath worked with more bands after that, and fashion jobs followed, along with a collaborative friendship with *i-D*'s young fashion editor at the time, Edward Enninful (now editor-in-chief of British *Vogue*).

Since then McGrath has created the make-up for hundreds of fashion shows and is a key part of the creative teams of photographers including Steven Meisel and Paolo Roversi. Her make-up can bring a fashion look to life, adding spirit, character and sparkle to any story.

In true entrepreneurial style, McGrath launched her make-up line, Pat McGrath Labs, independently, and her first product, the limited-edition Gold 001, sold out in no time. Cleopatra would surely have been first in the queue.

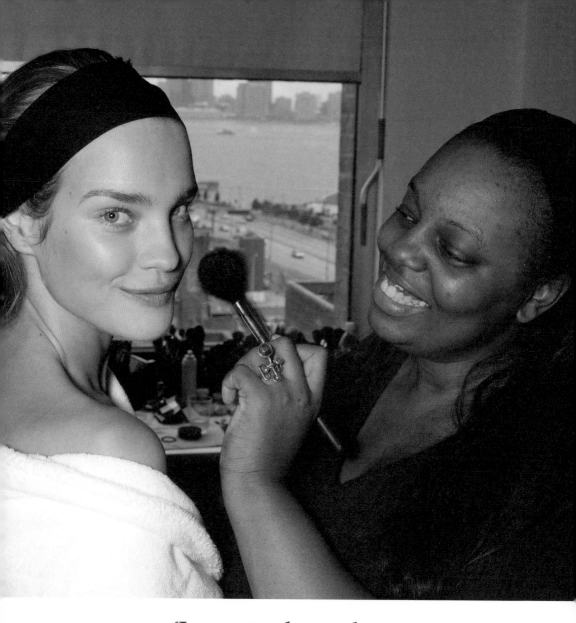

'I want to change how
people think about make-up,
and disrupt the status quo.'

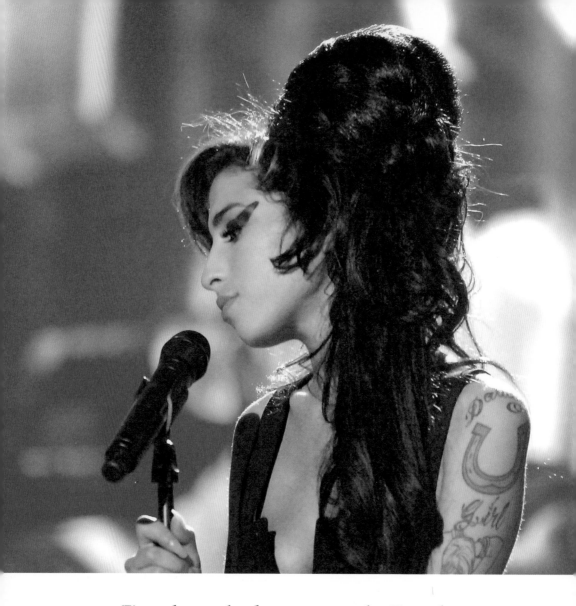

'I've always had my own style, I've always been different. I don't like to wear anything that anyone else is wearing because it's very important for me to make a statement.'

AMY WINEHOUSE

UK, 1983–2011

A my Winehouse, just 1.6 m (5 ft 3 in), with her matted mass of black backcombed hair, retro 1960s liquid eyeliner, consciously trashy style and satin ballet pumps, was every bit the Cleopatra. The north London daughter of a taxi driver, she was a powerful communicator and storyteller who took her cues, both musically and stylistically, from the jazz singers of the 1950s – Sarah Vaughan and Dinah Washington – and the teen-angst girl groups of the 1960s, particularly the Ronettes (see page 172). But her combination of unvarnished urban poetry, Camden Town vintage fashion, beehive hair and angry attitude was unique.

Winehouse's debut album, *Frank* (2003), spoke to a generation of women and men whose lives didn't always go as they were supposed to. She was honest about her own helter-skelter existence: she called out the men who had left her broken and down; she sang about rehab; she had no secrets and no shame. Her music spoke of her struggle with poor mental health, her drug addiction and a string of disastrous relationships.

By the time of the release of *Back to Black* in 2006, Winehouse had become a full-blown superstar. As her fame and confidence as a performer and songwriter grew, so did her style, which was always unashamedly rough around the edges and nostalgic for the days of 1950s jazz clubs. Sometimes she wore flowers in her hair, Billie Holiday-style, and at others cocktail umbrellas or a bandana. She was unpolished, a cross between the cartoon character Betty Boop and 1950s pin-ups (both of which she had as tattoos): big hair, pneumatic cleavage, cinched waist, short skirts.

Winehouse's shocking death at the age of 27 was a tragic waste of a phenomenal talent. The *New York Times* added her to 'a lineage of bad girls, extending from Cleopatra to Louise Brooks's Lulu to Salt-n-Pepa, irresistible man traps who always seem to come to the same unfortunate end'. Her music and her larger-than-life image will never be forgotten.

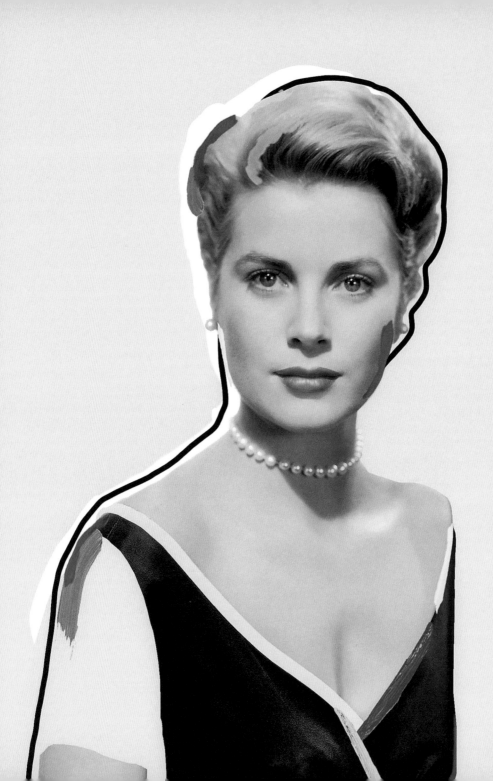

Blue Bloods

Some of us fantasized about being a princess when we grew up – or of marrying into royalty. For most of us it was just a phase, and soon enough we realized that there's much more to life than Disney gowns and tiaras. But for some, it's a birthright. And for a privileged few, a royal wedding is the dream that becomes reality.

WALLIS SIMPSON

Duchess of Windsor, USA, 1896–1986

'It lifts your morale to put on something different. Clothes are, after all, either a pep pill or a depressant.'

The royal family and the British public may have turned their backs on Wallis Simpson, but the fashion world did not. The twice-divorced American who stole Edward VIII's heart, resulting in his abdication from the throne, was the dream client. After all, she believed a woman could not be too rich or too thin, making her perfectly qualified to shop at the world's most exclusive couture houses.

The king's decision in December 1936 to renounce the throne to be with the woman he loved shook the British establishment. His brother Bertie replaced him, as George VI, and Edward and Wallis were cast off into a life of idle luxury. With no meaningful occupation or children, Simpson had little to do but ensure that she was the best-dressed woman in Paris. As she said: 'You have no idea how hard it is to live out a great romance.' Her friend Diana Vreeland (see page 36) described her as 'soignée, not degagée', which is to say smart, not casual. Slouch was not part of her vocabulary.

Simpson devoted herself to daily appointments with the hairdresser Alexandre de Paris (for a precise centre parting and an elaborate chignon that were copied by women worldwide) and endless rounds of dress fittings for social engagements, each one an opportunity to show off her latest purchase. She loved clothes and dressing up above all else, particularly pieces by Madeleine Vionnet, Elsa Schiaparelli (most famously the Lobster dress she wore to be photographed by Cecil Beaton for *Vogue*, before her marriage in 1937) and Dior. For Edward's funeral in 1972, she wore a precisely tailored dress by Hubert de Givenchy, who is said to have spent the night before the funeral perfecting the length of her chiffon veil. A tragic figure, her tiny frame immaculately turned out, she returned to Paris with nobody left to impress.

Wallis Simpson continues to inspire. Even though she was the scourge of the British royal family, the fashion designer Daniella Helayel (then of Issa) said she was thinking of Simpson's pale 'Wallis blue' wedding dress by Mainbocher when she made Kate Middleton's engagement dress in 2010. Ralph Lauren has paid homage too. And there was a flurry of designer excitement when Simpson was played by Andrea Riseborough in Madonna's film *W.E.* in 2011. The costumes were the real stars of the show, lovingly re-created in the spirit of Wallis by Arianne Phillips and sparking interest in Simpson's style and story for an entirely new generation.

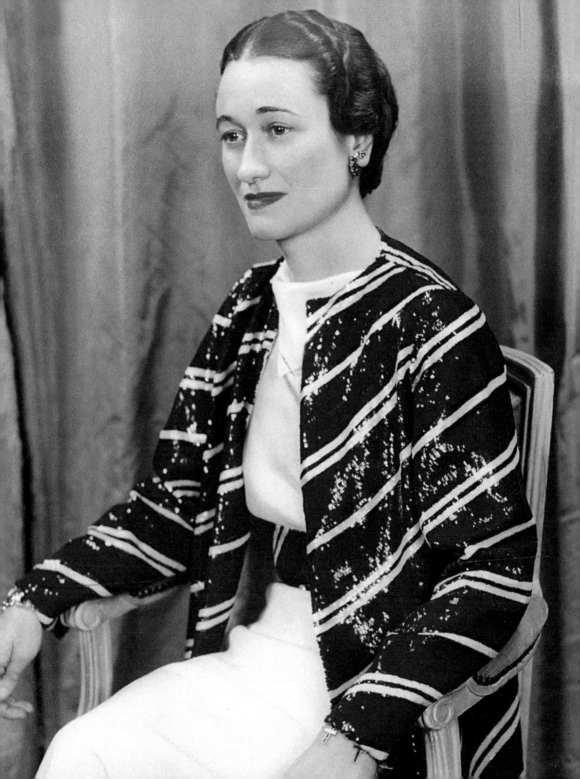

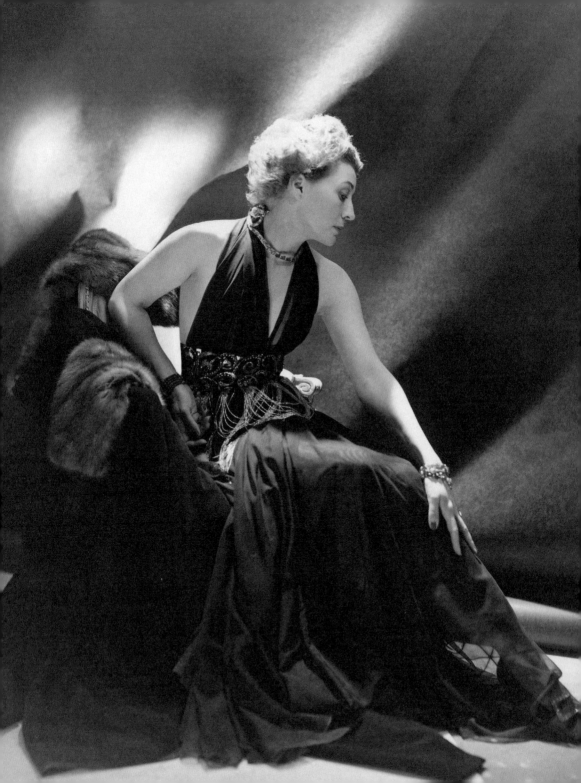

MONA VON BISMARCK

USA, 1897–1983

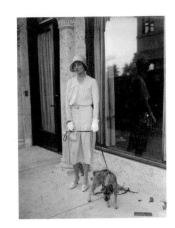

'Her life is worthy of a novel with all things beautiful'.

Hubert de Givenchy

Mona von Bismarck was a southern belle who married well – over and over again. Five times, in fact, making her well-travelled (her first honeymoon was spent on board her new husband Harrison Williams's boat *Warrior*, at the time the biggest, most glamorous yacht in the world); wealthy beyond most people's dreams; a respected hostess; a countess (thanks to husband number four, Count Albrecht Edzard Heinrich Karl von Bismarck-Schönhausen, grandson of the German chancellor Otto von Bismarck); and one of the twentieth century's most prolific consumers of art and fashion. Her friend the photographer Cecil Beaton described her as 'one of the few outstanding beauties of the thirties'. The jury is out on whether she had a heart of gold, or was a gold-digging social climber who abandoned her only son to her first husband in return for half a million dollars in alimony.

Bismarck's villa Il Fortino in Capri became a cornerstone of high society, and there she entertained everyone from the Duke and Duchess of Windsor (see page 184), Winston Churchill and Maria Callas to the great fashion editor Diana Vreeland (see page 36), who was at the villa in 1968 to relay the news that Bismarck's beloved couturier Balenciaga had closed shop, and reported that Mona did not leave her room for three days afterwards.

Bismarck's style trademarks, much imitated by her friends and by society influencers of the time, included colourless nail varnish (so chic), double-strand pearls, halter necks to show off her enviably athletic physique, cocktail pyjamas (why not?) and silver-grey hair. She favoured rooms decorated entirely in white and is said to have been the inspiration for the columnist Igor Cassini when he coined the phrase 'jet set'. Her fabulous clothes were so important to her that, when she commissioned Salvador Dalí to paint her portrait in 1943 and he provocatively painted her without them, she refused to pay for the work until he put some clothes on her. She had been voted best-dressed woman in 1933 by the French couture elite, after all. Dalí's only compromise was to put her in a dark, ragged shroud. After distributing her incredible fashion collection among various prestigious institutions, including the Victoria and Albert Museum, before her death, she was buried in a black and pink couture gown by Hubert de Givenchy. Fabulous.

DEBORAH CAVENDISH

Duchess of Devonshire, UK, 1920–2014

The late Duchess of Devonshire claimed not to be interested in politics (unlike her sister Unity, who was obsessed with Adolf Hitler and shot herself when Britain declared war on Germany), said she didn't read books apart from those by Beatrix Potter (although it was suspected that she had a secret reading habit, and she wrote several books herself), and was more interested in her garden and looking after her hens than in going to fashion shows. The youngest of the Mitford sisters, the six famous and sometimes notorious women who included Nancy the novelist, Unity the Fascist and Jessica the communist, Deborah was bullied by her siblings as a child. Nancy, the eldest, called her Nine, referring to the mental age she believed Deborah (or Debo, as she was known) had attained.

Debo excelled at country pursuits, however, and was allowed to start hunting at the precocious age of 12. She dreamed of marrying a duke, but ultimately became a duchess only by accident. She married Lord Andrew Cavendish, a second son, and it was only after his older brother was killed in action during World War II and his father, the duke, died in 1950 that they inherited the 297-room Chatsworth House in Derbyshire and Deborah found her calling – as its chatelaine. She made it her life's work to restore the house, gardens and farm to create a thriving, sustainable business.

Debo had a wonderfully dry sense of humour and a passion for Elvis Presley, hated city life and collected insect and spider brooches. She exemplified a certain eccentric tweedy English country look, and her apparent lack of interest in the traditional trappings of the fashionable elite was part of her wonderful charm. When Bruce Weber photographed her, he recalled, 'she had this really beautiful dress that was made especially for her by Jean Patou. She said, "I think it'd be nice to wear it feeding my chickens." I don't think that there's ever been a more elegant woman photographed feeding chickens.'

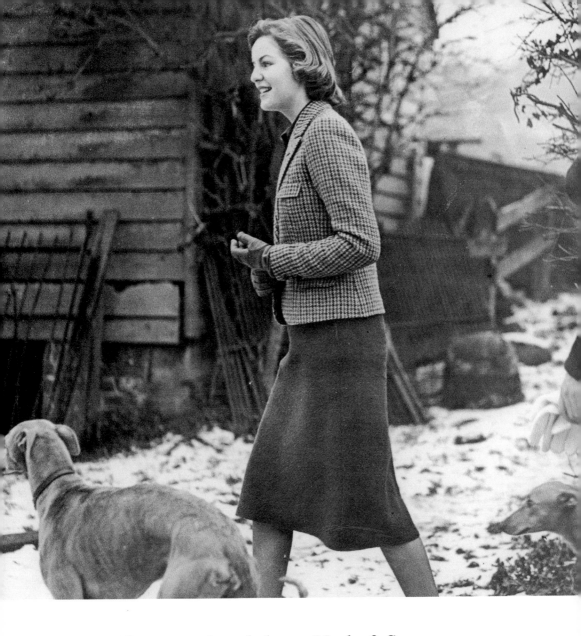

'After agricultural shows, Marks & Spencer
is the place to go shopping, and then Paris.
Nothing in between seems to be much good.'

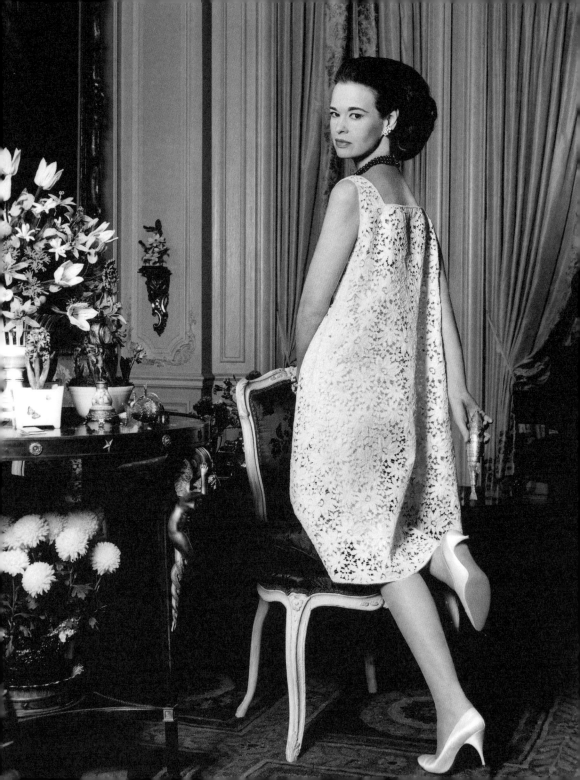

GLORIA VANDERBILT

USA, born 1924

'The fame you earn has a different taste from the fame that is forced upon you.'

When Gloria Vanderbilt was first photographed by Louise Dahl-Wolfe for *Harper's Bazaar* in 1939, she was just 15. Born into one of America's wealthiest families (the Vanderbilts were railway magnates), she had dark eyes and pale skin, inherited from her Chilean great-grandmother, and this teenager had just designed an Egypt-themed room at her aunt's house.

Vanderbilt's original sense of style is almost as extraordinary as her life story. At the age of 17, when she was visiting her estranged mother in Los Angeles, the film director Howard Hughes romanced her on his private jet. An endless stream of men, including Marlon Brando and Frank Sinatra, fell in love with this unfathomably glamorous young woman.

Vanderbilt's style was inspirational and celebrated, from the 'table dresses' designed by Howard Greer (he specialized in dresses that were a sensation from the waist up) and the Mainbocher hostess dresses of the mid-1960s, to the extraordinary patchwork dress made for her by the Cuban couturier Adolfo, which was on the moodboard for the Valentino collection in 2015. Richard Avedon photographed her throughout her life, documenting her collection of Fortuny dresses for American *Vogue* in 1969.

An actor, painter, writer and fashion designer – she launched her own line of jeans in 1974 at Studio 54 in New York, selling six million pairs in the first year – Vanderbilt also became known for her exuberant collage decoration techniques. For a woman who was born into untold wealth, she is a restless and powerful creative force. From textiles and ceramics to greetings cards, sunglasses and bed linen, she was one of the first great personality lifestyle brands. In 2017, at the age of 93, she joined Instagram, sharing pictures of her colourful life and work. Her sheer determination to be someone on her own terms became her greatest strength. In 1970 her last husband, the film writer Wyatt Cooper, wrote: 'If she has not made of herself a living work of art, she's come damned close, or as close as anybody I'd ever want to meet.'

JACQUELINE KENNEDY ONASSIS

USA, 1929–1994

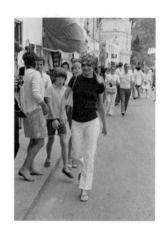

*'I am a woman above
everything else.'*

As First Lady of the United States between 1961 and 1963, Jacqueline Kennedy was scrutinized by the eyes of the world – each outfit, every subtle change of hairstyle, the length of her gloves, the colour of her coats, the idealized perfection of her life. During her first year in the White House, she famously spent $45,446 more on her wardrobe than her husband's annual $100,000 salary as president. Much of it went on the couture outfits made for her by Oleg Cassini, and she was also enamoured of the French couturiers Chanel, Balenciaga and Givenchy.

The 'Jackie look' has been copied ever since. It was a simple silhouette: boxy jacket, matching neat, A-line skirt cut to the knee, coat worn over the top echoing the shape. Kim Kardashian didn't come close when she was photographed in Kennedy style for *Interview* magazine in 2017, showing that style is more than simply the clothes you wear.

Kennedy liked pastel colours, and neutral beige and fawn. She was bold in her strapless evening gowns, usually in a low heel designed by her friend Hélène Arpels. She popularized the pillbox hat, which, made by the designer Halston, added a military formality to everything she wore. She set the tone for a generation of women who strove for the same control and perfection in the way they dressed and lived their lives.

After John F. Kennedy's assassination, Jackie did not change out of her blood-stained pink Chanel suit for the swearing-in of President Lyndon B. Johnson aboard Air Force One. The bloodied suit became symbolic of a time of violent and political turmoil in the United States.

For her marriage five years later to the shipping magnate Aristotle Onassis, Jackie wore a suitably demure, high-necked, knee-length number in ivory lace with luxurious bell sleeves and a pleated skirt. It was made by Valentino, the designer to the Mediterranean fashion elite. Jackie's style loosened up to fit her new jet-set, sun-drenched life, and she continued to influence women in her choice of silk shirts, cool hipster slacks, designer logo belts and, of course, her slouchy Gucci handbag. Nicknamed 'Jackie O', she was pursued even more by the paparazzi, and although she continued to wear the glamorous, oversized bug-eyed sunglasses that were part of her signature, along with headscarves, she failed splendidly ever to look remotely anonymous.

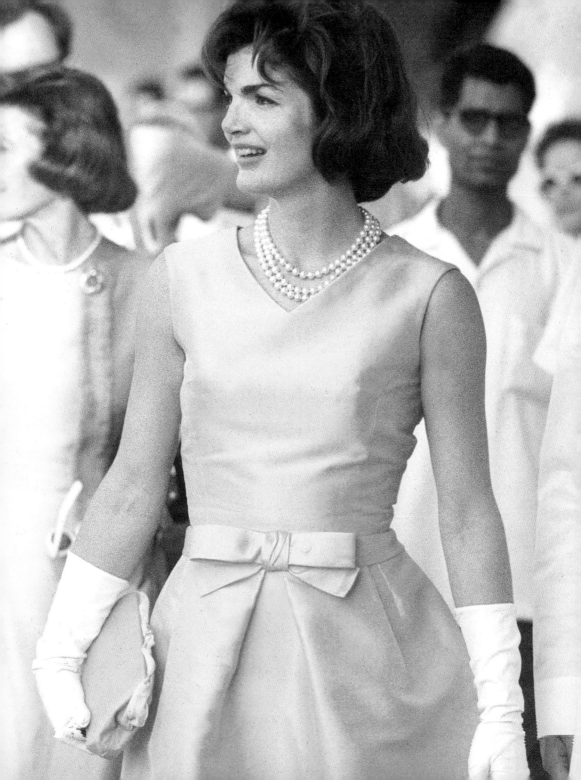

GRACE KELLY

USA, 1929–1982

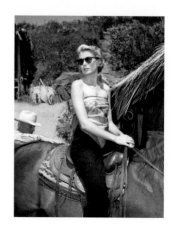

'I favour pearls on-screen and in my private life.'

In March 1955 Grace Kelly arrived at the Academy Awards ceremony in a floor-length gown of palest aquamarine duchess satin with exquisitely turned rouleaux straps that crossed on each shoulder. With it she wore a cloak, pastel-blue slippers and elbow-length gloves in pristine white. Her hair looked like freshly spun golden silk. Up against Audrey Hepburn and Judy Garland for Best Actress, Kelly did not expect to win, but when she set foot on the stage to receive her award (for *The Country Girl*) there was really no contest. For many women, she has remained the gold standard, the timeless fashion star.

That Oscars dress was designed by Hollywood's leading wardrobe mistress, Edith Head, who said Kelly knew how to wear good-quality, expensive clothes because she had been a model. Certainly, Kelly's wardrobe in *Rear Window* (1954), also designed by Head, is a lesson in perfectly stated luxurious elegance, a touch Ivy League prep, a touch high-class debutante. She could even make jeans and a pair of penny loafers look like perfection. Pause at any frame of that film and your wardrobe will thank you for it.

As well as having a frame and height that made her the ideal clothes horse for costume designers (at

1.69 m/5ft 6½ in, she was taller than many of her leading men), Kelly had impeccable, classic taste off-screen. She exuded quiet confidence whether she was wearing a ballgown, a shirt and capri pants, a skirt suit or a silk dress, often with a string of pearls round her neck. She was given the ultimate accolade when the Hermès bag she carried in *To Catch a Thief* (1955) was named after her, ensuring ongoing waiting lists for an accessory that symbolizes style and class.

Kelly's wedding to Prince Rainier III of Monaco in 1956 involved 25 m (82 ft) of silk taffeta and 125-year-old Brussels rose-point lace (which inspired the Duchess of Cambridge's wedding dress in 2011) and was watched on television by 30 million people. Her transformation from Hollywood icon to heroine of a real-life fairy tale was complete. In return, she gave up her Hollywood career. When Alfred Hitchcock invited her to make a comeback as the lead in his film *Marnie* (1964; the role was ultimately taken by Tippi Hedren) the prince did not allow her to do so, but she remained the famous director's dream leading lady. She continues as inspiration for the eternal icy blonde, from January Jones's character in *Mad Men* to Gwyneth Paltrow.

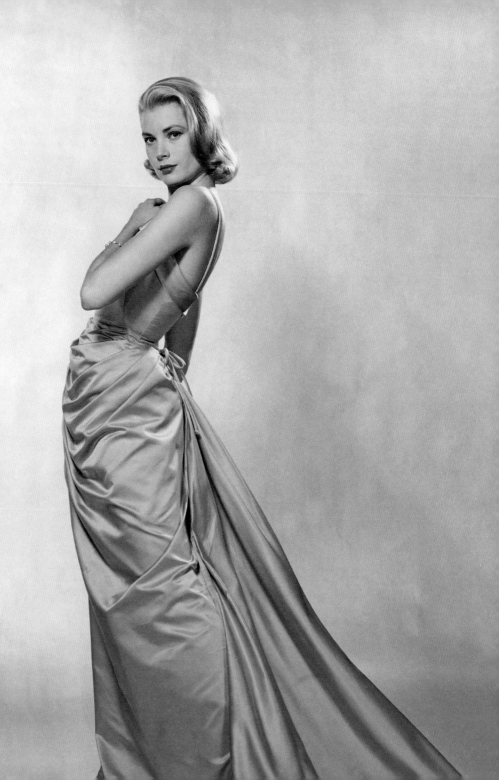

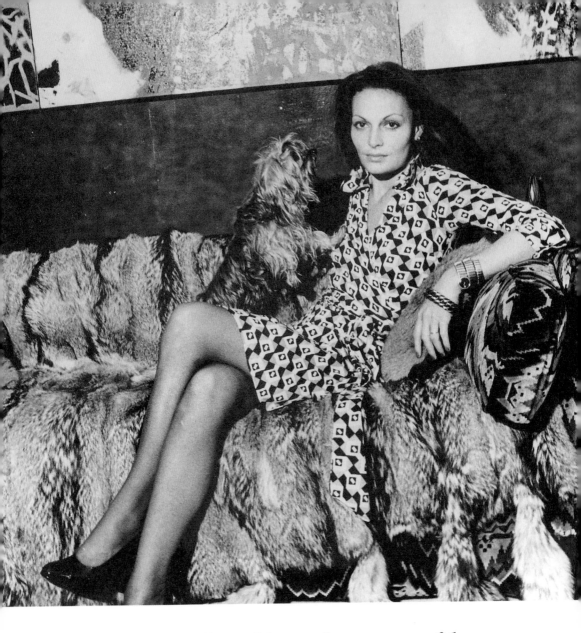

'I really sell confidence, because confidence
is what allows you to design your life and
be the person you are or want to be.'

DIANE VON FURSTENBERG

Belgium, born 1946

Diane von Furstenberg, the American designer and one-time princess who launched her business in 1974 on the back of a simple idea – the wrap dress – that became a design classic almost overnight, loves to give advice. Her girlfriends – from the Russian supermodel and philanthropist Natalia Vodianova to Naomi Campbell (see page 21) – are of all ages and she is somehow ageless among them, a mother figure, an older sister, the coolest girl in the class. One of her dresses has even been acquired by the Smithsonian Institution in Washington, DC, as part of its permanent collection of design classics.

If you've ever worn one of Furstenberg's famous wrap dresses (or even one of the endless copies they have inspired), you will have felt the warm glow of DVF too. She observed that when Madonna (see page 51) needed to look smart and businesslike, she did so in a DVF dress. The style is universal in its appeal, fitting a wide range of body shapes and updated each season in a variety of prints and patterns.

Furstenberg is very much the product of her upbringing. Her parents were Jewish émigrés who survived the Holocaust. Her mother spent 13 months in Auschwitz from the age of 19, after being caught working for the Belgian resistance. Despite her frail state, she gave birth to a daughter the year after the war ended. It's amazing to consider what this daughter went on to achieve as a designer and a business-woman, presiding over a global brand worth $200 million.

Furstenberg's business ambition has been matched by her two glittering marriages. With her first husband, the German prince Egon von Fürstenberg, she moved to New York in the early 1970s, and they became one of the disco era's most celebrated couples, part of the Andy Warhol art and glamour set. Since 2001 she has been married to the media tycoon Barry Diller. A woman with less drive and passion might have been tempted to put her feet up or spend her days organizing charity fundraisers, but Furstenberg is on a mission. She has well and truly made her mark, but every time a woman wears one of her dresses she spreads a little more confidence.

INÈS DE LA FRESSANGE

France, born 1957

Even when she started modelling, at the age of 19, Inès de La Fressange was more of a personality than a conventional clothes horse. Not that she didn't look great in anything any designer cared to throw at her; with her lanky, self-confessed 'green-bean' 1.8 m (5 ft 11 in) figure, she was born to model. But she would treat the catwalk as a social event, often stopping to greet someone she knew in the audience or pulling silly faces. She didn't take it seriously, and her nonchalance is precisely what made her so attractive. It's an ebullience that she inherited from her mother, the Argentinian beauty Cecilia Sánchez-Cirez, also a model, who married the noble but bohemian André de Seignard, Marquis de La Fressange.

Inès herself ended up having a close relationship with the house of Chanel. She was a regular on the Chloé catwalk when Karl Lagerfeld was designing the collections in the 1970s, and when he took over at Chanel in 1983, he asked La Fressange to join him as the face of the brand. A dream brand ambassador, she breathed her fabulous, Gauloise-y breath into the house. With her sparkling smile and chic shrug, she helped to revive Chanel for a new generation who aspired to the way she wore her tweed suit with piles of pearl necklaces, a jaunty hat, a cheeky grin and a cigarette on the go at all times. And if you couldn't afford Chanel, you wore the Kookaï rip-off – but in your mind you were still Inès, swinging your gilt-chained bag and hailing a taxi on the Champs-Elysées.

As La Fressange has got older, she has only become more confident in her own boyish, effortless style. She has a wonderfully democratic approach to fashion: she always knows where to find a bargain, and will happily mix a T-shirt from the French discount department store Tati with a pair of Roger Vivier heels. Thankfully, now that La Fressange is designing collections for Uniqlo, everyone can possess a touch of her particular brand of French *je ne sais quoi*.

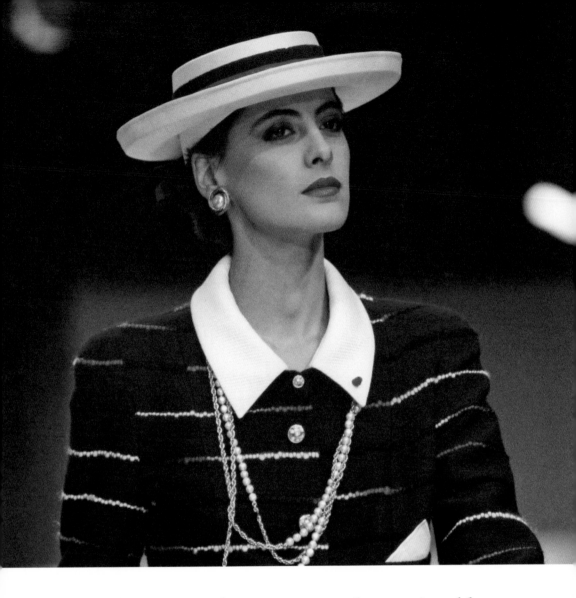

'Nothing gives the impression that you're old
more than being obsessed by looking young.
It's very ugly when women refuse to get old.'

DIANA, PRINCESS OF WALES

UK, 1961–1997

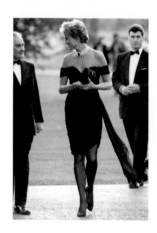

With girly pie-crust collars, tweedy skirts, patterned cardis, everyday jeans and, of course, that hair and shy, crooked smile, Diana Spencer was the ultimate Sloane Ranger, and the cover girl of Ann Barr and Peter York's *Official Sloane Ranger Handbook* (1982). This posh subcult was the very antithesis of the working-class punk that was so incongruously happening at the same time. By the time she became Princess of Wales, she had redefined the look and made it her own: the pie-crust collars had become full-on ruffles and frills; the velvet ribbon neckties had evolved into grand pussy bows; the shoulder pads had become more pronounced. There were sailor suits, and there was weekend country attire – corduroy trousers and statement Peruvian jumpers. Diana had transformed herself from slightly frumpy nursery teacher to one of the most influential style icons of all time (and I use the word 'icon' most reservedly, even in a book about icons).

As the 'People's Princess', Diana had something that touched those who weren't usually in awe of royalty. She did it in many ways, primarily through her work supporting people with HIV and AIDS at a time when that was a taboo and much-misunderstood subject. But one of her primary methods of communication was the way she dressed. Her clothes, her make-up, her shoes, her accessories and her innate style were her toolkit, and she played with them all unreservedly. The famous image of her sitting on her own in front of the Taj Mahal, the most potent symbol of love and loneliness, was given all the more impact by her choice of colourful, graphic clothes. The short, off-the-shoulder body-con dress and heels she wore on the evening of the summer party at the Serpentine Gallery in London in 1994 – the night Prince Charles admitted his infidelity with Camilla Parker Bowles in an interview on the ITV network – was a showstopper, an 'Up yours' to an ex-lover, a refusal to be downtrodden by a failed relationship.

Diana's impact on the way we dress continues, from the soulful, smudgy eye make-up to the sporty athleisure wear, the 1980s Sloaney pie crusts and her cool way with a white shirt and khakis. She was the ultimate fairy-tale princess who used her clothes to tell her story.

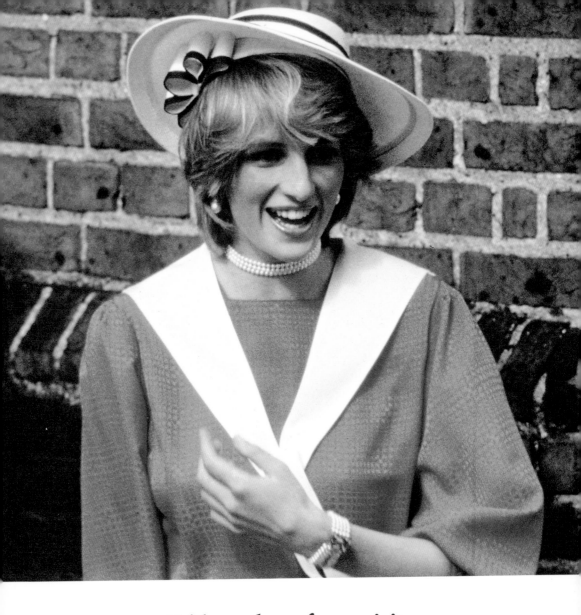

'I like to be a free spirit.
Some don't like that, but
that's the way I am.'

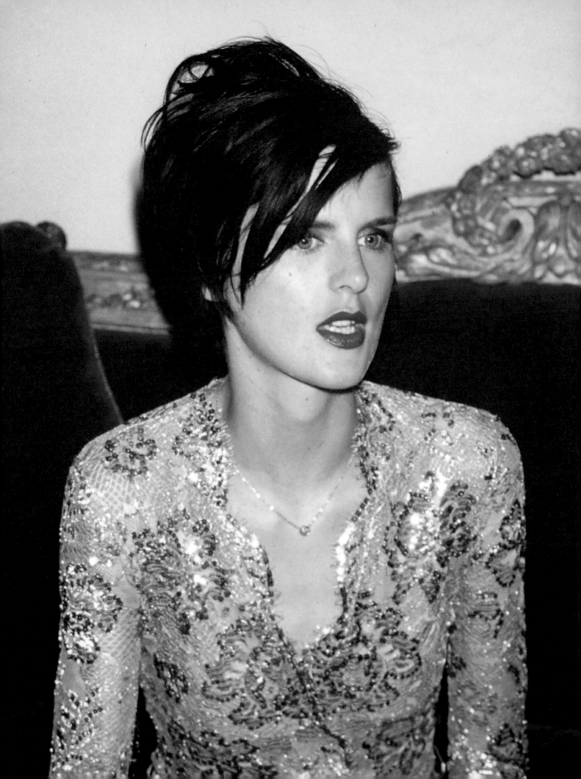

STELLA TENNANT

UK, born 1970

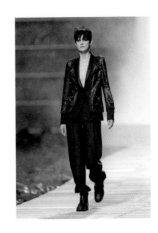

'I don't think of myself as kind of a classic beauty.'

It was the nose ring that did it. When she first appeared in British *Vogue* in 1993 as part of Steven Meisel's now famous 'Anglo-Saxon Attitudes' shoot, Stella Tennant had an upper-crust haughtiness and wilful boyishness that were unsettling. She had just finished her sculpture degree at Winchester School of Art, and the fashion matchmaker Isabella Blow (see page 52) had asked if she would like to be photographed by Meisel. 'He didn't want to work with people who were models,' she said in an interview for *VideoFashion* in 2012. 'He wanted to work with normal people. So, I'm not really a normal person any more, but I was then.'

Tennant had had her nose and navel pierced in June 1993, and started modelling the following month as a way of contradicting assumptions people might make about her. 'The nose ring definitely makes people remember me,' she told the *New York Times* fashion critic Amy Spindler in October that year. London was the centre of Britpop, a new wave in art, music and fashion, and Tennant, with her rebellious aristocratic looks, was the embodiment of the scene at that time. She was properly posh – the granddaughter of the Duchess of Devonshire (see page 188) – and had grown up on a large sheep farm in Scotland. But she was no passive debutante. She refused to smile, and made a speciality of looking seriously pissed-off as she stomped up and down the catwalk. In the early 1990s Tennant was a regular model for Helmut Lang, and in 1999 she was married in a white knee-length vest dress by him.

Tennant's magic lay in the fact that she was so much part of the fashion world – the face of Chanel, no less – while also keeping a healthy distance from it with her real life back home in the Scottish countryside. She is a role model for a certain kind of girl who loves fashion and self-expression but is determined to do things her way, to stand out as an individual and to break all the rules.

MEGHAN, DUCHESS OF SUSSEX

USA, born 1981

'I'm still the same person that I am, and I've never defined myself by my relationship.'

Not since Diana, Princess of Wales (see page 200), has a member of the British royal family had such a colossal impact on the world. But the image of Meghan Markle on her wedding day, immaculately dressed in luminous white Givenchy, was immediately the stuff of fashion legend. The simplicity of the veil, with its representations of the countries of the Commonwealth, was a symbol, if not quite of equality, then at least of solidarity with people around the world. The new Duchess of Sussex is, after all, a 'commoner', an ordinary citizen (albeit a television personality), and her biracial heritage suddenly made the British royal family relevant, inclusive and above all modern.

No wonder, then, that whatever Meghan wears is watched with fervid anticipation, every stitch and seam dissected by the fashion press; every outfit copied by her fans; every hairstyle, handbag, shoe and accessory digested by the high street, to be included in the next collection. It's called the 'Meghan effect': a black 'Jackie O' dress by Black Halo sold out within hours after she was seen wearing it.

As an actor, Meghan is familiar with the idea of using clothes to create a character, and she has admitted to borrowing clothes from Rachel Zane, her character in the American television show *Suits*. Like Diana before her, she is acutely aware of the messages her clothes send. Her choice of a female designer – the recently appointed Clare Waight Keller at Givenchy – to create her wedding dress was no accident. Having lived in Los Angeles, she has been at the epicentre of the #TimesUp campaign, acutely aware of the new feminism that she feels a responsibility to champion. Likewise, her choice of Stella McCartney – the queen of more conscious ethical fashion (see page 160) – to design her evening wedding dress signified a more thoughtful approach to her wardrobe.

In her own fashion choices, Meghan leans strongly towards the classic style of Audrey Hepburn, Jackie Kennedy Onassis and Grace Kelly (see pages 122, 192 and 194), favouring clean, elegant lines. In her role as a duchess she has quickly found a wardrobe for a woman who works rather than a lady who lunches.

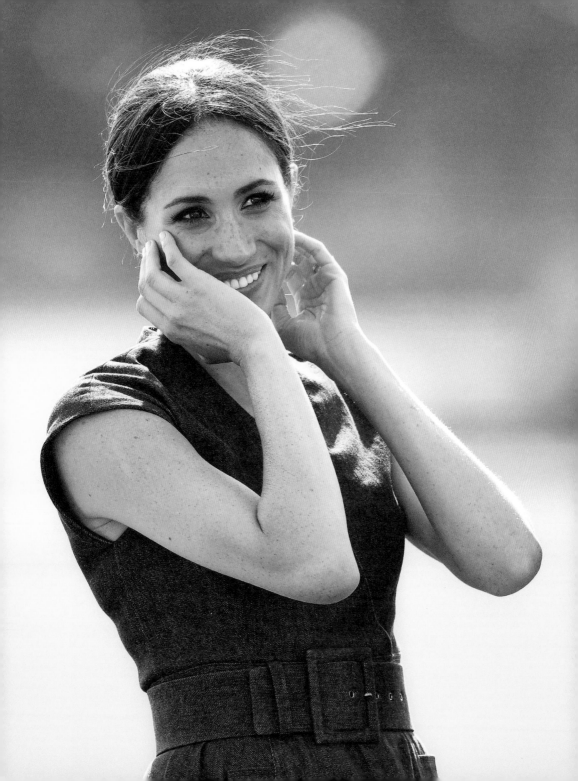

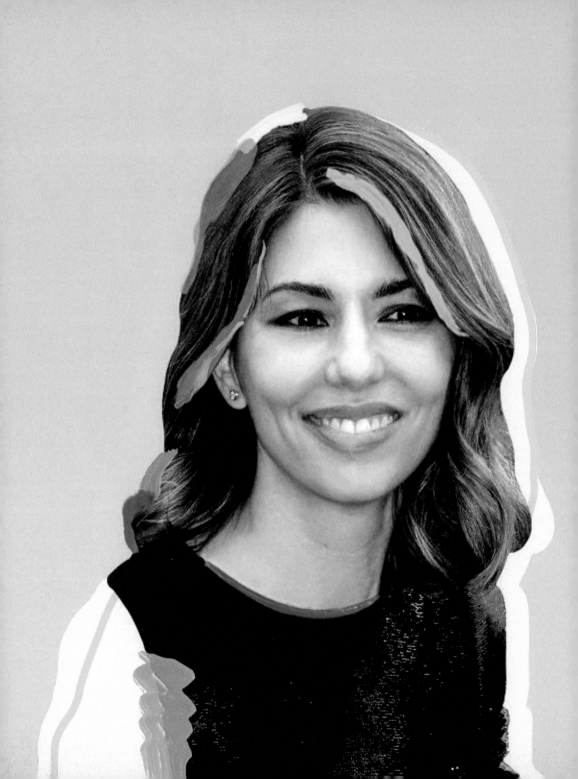

Girl
Crushes

Who's your girl crush? You know, the girl
you're secretly a little in love with, slightly
older, slightly wiser, slightly better dressed
than you. She's the girl you'd like to be,
whose hair you want and whose entire
wardrobe would be your dressing-up
dream come true.

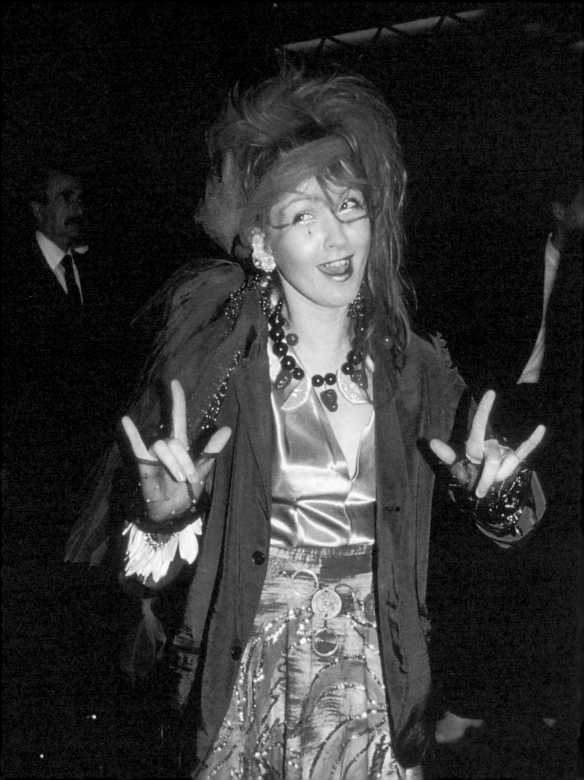

CYNDI LAUPER

USA, born 1953

'I think it's just fun to look different.'

Cyndi Lauper was the crazy, zany, feminist face of 1980s pop. While Madonna (see page 51) was cool, sexy and a little risqué, Lauper was the one you would actually have liked to go out with on a wild girls' night out, a blur of backcombed, crazily coloured hair, a flurry of net underskirts and a jangle of earrings. She bounced about like a pogo stick, pulled silly faces, broke all the rules of the colour wheel and didn't care a jot what anyone thought of her.

But Lauper's message was far deeper than her slapstick performances might have suggested, as the title of her debut album, *She's so Unusual* (1983), suggests. She wasn't a typical pop star. She was never interested in being stereotypically sexy, but rather in breaking down barriers – particularly those of gender inequality. For her, pop was political. In 1983 she rewrote the lyrics of Robert Hazard's 'Girls Just Wanna Have Fun',

which was originally written from a male perspective. The video begins with her arguing with her mother at home in the kitchen, and then gathering her multiracial, ambisexual mix of friends with everyone she meets along the way, from stuffy businessmen to construction workers, for a party in her room. Just for a moment, she has said, it was the straight guy who was the odd one out.

At a time when Ronald Reagan and Margaret Thatcher were in charge, when battles over equality and sexuality were still being fought and a generation was being threatened by the horror of AIDS, Lauper's song had a powerful impact. A decade before the Spice Girls, she sang about sexual equality and unfettered girl power. Girls – and many boys, too – wanted to have fun, and the freedom to dress and behave as they liked.

SADE ADU

Nigeria, born 1959

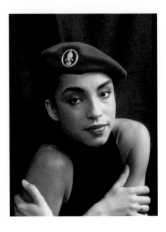

'If the house was on fire, I wouldn't leave until I was fully made up.'

Why do so many people have a crush on Sade Adu? Is it the perfectly slicked-back waist-length ponytail? The oversized gold hooped earrings? The red lips? The seductive sweep of the eyes? The batwing sleeves? When she seared her way on to our television screens in 1984, she was cool, confident, smoky and sleek in black mohair, singing 'Your Love Is King'. She was already too hip for *Top of the Pops*.

As part of the Saint Martin's School of Art group, Sade specialized in designing menswear and hung out with the music/art/fashion set. Her boyfriend at the time was the music journalist Robert Elms, and the couple was at the epicentre of London's in-crowd.

The thing about Sade is that she always knew she was different. Her English mother and Nigerian father had met in London but married and moved to Nigeria, and she was born in Ibidan, Nigeria's third-largest city. She was christened Helen Folasade Adu, but her Nigerian family called her Sade. Her parents split up when she was four, and she moved to Colchester,

Essex, with her mother and older brother – the only two black kids on her estate. At the age of 18, Sade moved to London to live in a converted fire station and study fashion at Saint Martin's, hoping she could learn a trade and earn a living as a fashion designer. By the time she was singing backing vocals in her first band, Pride, her tough but sensual style was set – the long plait (with a blonde strand running through it), always with an eye for a killer accessory. She went on to form the band Sade with three other members of Pride, and together they have sold over 50 million records and are still making music.

Sade Adu's look perfectly reflected the laid-back jazz vibe of 1980s London: shades of Billie Holiday (see page 150), but with a modern edge. There is not a dud outfit in her entire career, from little black Lycra dresses to masculine white shirts worn with Levi's 501s, white jeans with loafers, nifty little bolero jackets for a Spanish look on 'The Sweetest Taboo' (1985) and a killer trench coat in 'When Am I Going to Make a Living?' (1984). She's a classic.

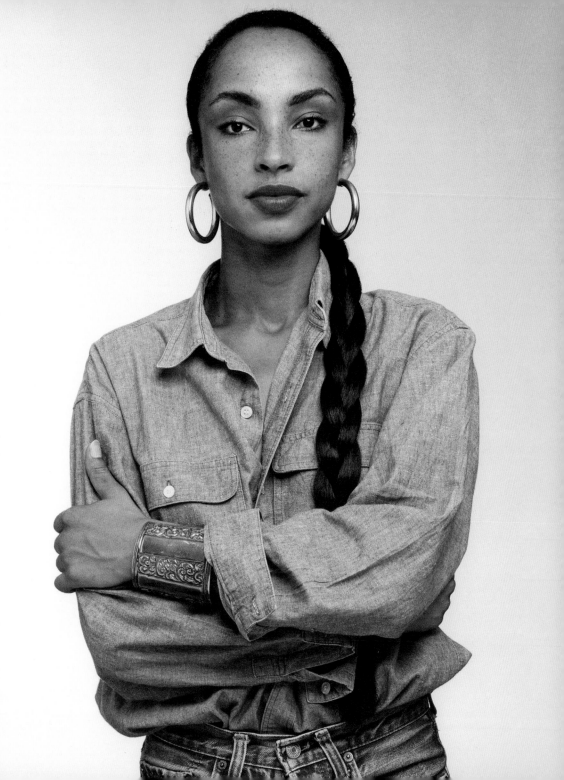

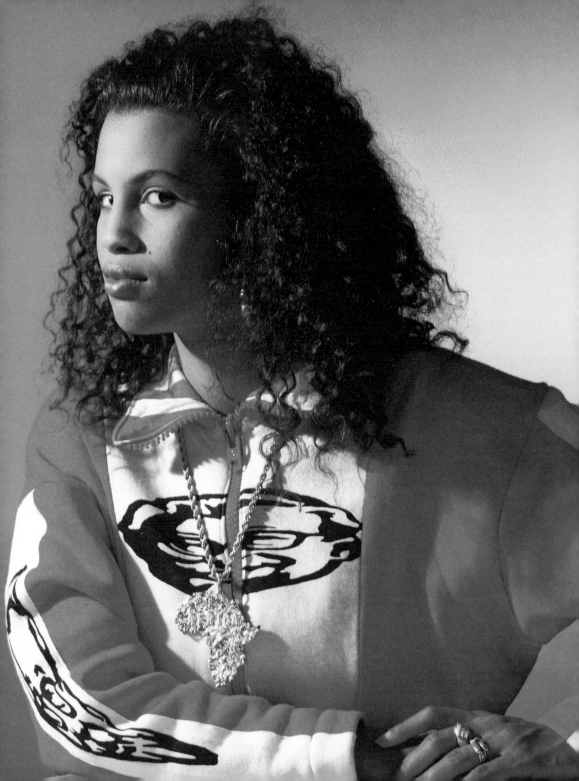

NENEH CHERRY

Sweden, born 1964

'I've never been very good at fitting into boxes.'

She's the Buffalo Girl. Neneh Cherry's first album, *Raw Like Sushi*, was a bestseller when it was released in 1989, and, in her orange bomber jacket, she perfectly captured the late 1980s moment with the hit single 'Buffalo Stance'. The stylist Ray Petri launched his 'Buffalo' look – which he described as 'a functional and stylish look; non-fashion with a hard attitude' – and Cherry was part of the gang. Their pictures became a regular fixture in *The Face* magazine. When she appeared on *Top of the Pops* seven months pregnant, she rapped her way through the song in body-hugging Lycra, oblivious to the way girl pop stars were supposed to look. She was earthy, sexy, hip, young, glorious.

Cherry had arrived in London in the 1970s at the age of 14. She was born in Stockholm, but her family also spent time in New York. She had been introduced to the punk band the Slits by her stepfather, the experimental jazz musician Don Cherry, and joined the band for a while, sharing a squat with the Slits singer, Ari Up (see page 69), before singing with the hugely influential early 1980s jazz punk band Rip Rig + Panic, dressed in a jumble of thrift-store clothes, African print dresses, colourful turbans and headscarves.

Cherry's style developed into a manifestation of the eighties style bible *The Face*: urban, street and slightly underground, complete with MA-1 flight jacket, high-top trainers, cycling shorts (remember those?), chunky hoop earrings and a huge gold dollar-sign medallion around her neck. It was New York hip hop and rap mixed with London art school, a good dose of punk DIY, customized Camden Market pick 'n' mix and Afrobeat. Her nomadic upbringing and raw energy were just an extra layer in this fertile melting pot of style and culture. She was helped on her way by her friend the stylist and jewellery designer Judy Blame, who was closely linked with the style press, *The Face* and *i-D*. Cherry was an inspiration to a whole new generation of hip-hop soul girls, including the duo Salt-N-Pepa, who were as serious about their music as they were about their style.

MOLLY RINGWALD

USA, born 1968

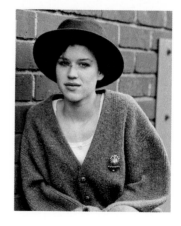

*'It did feel like the world
had a crush on me.'*

A nyone who has seen the Brat Pack films *The Breakfast Club* (1985) and *Pretty in Pink* (1986) will have a special place in their hearts for Molly Ringwald. She was the ultimate It girl of the decade, with her flame-red hair and perfectly sulky gloss-pink pout.

In her role as Claire in the cult teen movie *The Breakfast Club*, Ringwald was playing against type: rich, spoiled, horribly superficial – the girl at school everyone loved to hate. She brought a certain sophistication to the role, particularly in the wardrobe department. Instead of the stereotypical brash miniskirt and shoulder pads, her outfit was closer to something a smart city girl would wear: dusty pink V-neck T-shirt, mid-length pencil skirt in tweedy brown and knee-high leather boots. Her hair was blow-dried into a flicky bob, and she had diamond studs in her ears. She said she knew girls like that at her own school because 'there's no school without a girl like Claire Standish.'

As Andie in *Pretty in Pink*, Ringwald's look is part Sloane Ranger, part mad aunt, part hand-me down princess. She wins the prize for worst ever prom dress, a Pepto-Bismol-pink polka-dot concoction she whips up for herself out of a second-hand dress, all lace inserts and shoulder cut-outs. It's all she can afford, and she's proud of it. Andie's DIY nerdy thrift-store wardrobe – men's suit jackets mixed with granny cameo brooches at the collar, chintzy leggings, lacy collars, second-hand shoes, furnishing fabrics and pearls – defined the mid-1980s for countless women. She didn't care if she didn't get it right all the time. What mattered was her individuality and her strength of character. She was the outsider we all identified with.

In real life, Ringwald's style wasn't far removed from Andie's. For a while she dated Dweezil Zappa (son of the jazz musician Frank Zappa), who was the perfect match. She would wear a man's shirt with a colourful tie knotted at the neck and wire-rimmed specs perched on her nose, or a cable-knit jumper and big felt hat. She wasn't like other Hollywood starlets – but that's what made her the coolest girl of them all.

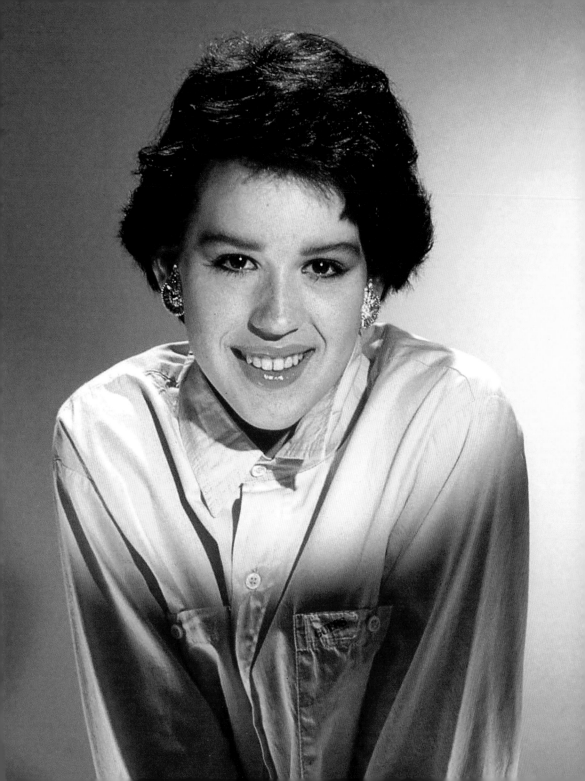

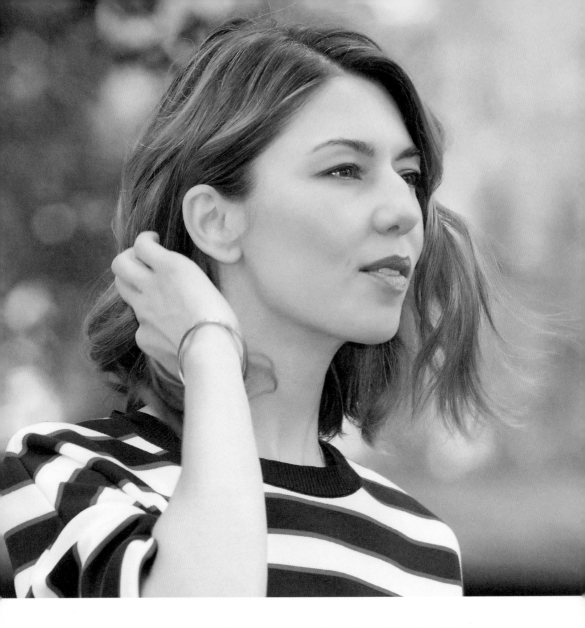

'You're considered superficial and silly if you are interested in fashion, but I think you can be substantial and still be interested in frivolity.'

SOFIA COPPOLA

USA, born 1971

She was born into Hollywood royalty and has become fashion royalty, too. As the daughter of the director Francis Ford Coppola, Sofia Coppola grew up on the sets of some of Hollywood's greatest movies. Her first screen appearance was as the baby Michael Francis Rizzi being baptized in *The Godfather* (1972). From that point a career in Hollywood seemed inevitable. In 1999 for her first film as director, *The Virgin Suicides*, she had a strong vision of how she thought Jeffrey Eugenides's book should look, and it was very different from the way teenage girls are usually portrayed in film. It was a pure, feminine vision – romantic, dreamy, white and light.

Since then, Coppola has made films with a strong female perspective, from the quirky *Lost in Translation* (2003) to *Marie Antoinette* (2006). For the latter, she used a highly stylized colour palette in all shades of the famous Ladurée macarons. The film influenced the next few seasons in fashion, resulting in a flurry of kitten heels, feather accessories, fans and bustiers.

Coppola's love of fashion runs hand in hand with her film-making, and you have only to look at her to see that she has exquisite taste. She never, ever looks as though she's tried too hard. In the mid-1990s she founded her own fashion label, Milkfed, with her friend Stephanie Hayman. It produced cool baby T-shirts printed with slogans such as 'Wasted' or an image of Che Guevara, shrunken nylon slip dresses and hipster trousers – the sort of thing Coppola and her friends Amanda de Cadenet and Zoe Cassavetes would wear to hang out at the well-known Hollywood retreat Chateau Marmont.

Coppola is great friends with Marc Jacobs and has been the face of his brand, as well as his muse while he was at Louis Vuitton. As she gets older her youthful, elegant style, choppy shoulder-length bob and unfussy approach to clothes evolve with her. She still loves to go to shows at New York Fashion Week, but she doesn't seem like a glossy celebrity interloper; she's just part of the scene.

CHLOË SEVIGNY

USA, born 1974

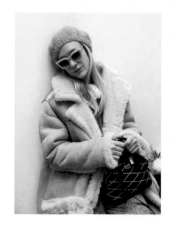

'Cool has a certain mystery to it. It's being removed. To me, the coolest thing is to keep something to yourself.'

In 1995 Chloë Sevigny starred as Jennie in a film written by her then boyfriend, Harmony Korine. They had met in the edgy Washington Square Park while she was at high school. *Kids*, directed by Larry Clark, was an instant cult hit, and her future as an uncompromisingly independent star was sealed.

Sevigny had already worked as an intern at *Sassy* magazine in New York, after one of its fashion editors spotted her on the street in a pair of corduroy overalls, but it was a feature in the *New Yorker* by Jay McInerney in 1994 that ensured her status as the coolest girl in the world. Everything she did was two steps ahead of the curve, from her jelly sandals to her second-hand 1980s Fila sweater. She grew up going thrift-store shopping with her mum, and was a fashion-magazine junkie who had a sixth sense when it came to spotting an Yves Saint Laurent dress. She is still a big fan of vintage clothes, and likes to mix those pieces with whatever else she is wearing.

Sevigny is one of those girls who simply have a natural instinct for what's cool. She's the girl who designers will watch and copy, and what she wears on the red carpet will appear on the high street the next month, so it made sense for her to design her own collections, with her friends Humberto Leon and Carol Lim of the cutting-edge fashion shop Opening Ceremony. She's kept most of her clothes in storage in Connecticut, where she grew up, forming an archive that most designers would kill for access to.

Sevigny is one of the few actors who has managed to keep her own style on the red carpet. She always looks as though she has dressed herself, rather than let a stylist pull together an outfit for her. For her role on the jury at the Cannes Film Festival in 2018, she wore mostly Chanel but sprinkled in some of her own pieces, some vintage Levi's, some Y/Project, always careful to make each look her own. She's an inspiration for all other free spirits to trust their own instincts and be themselves. That, ultimately, is the coolest thing possible.

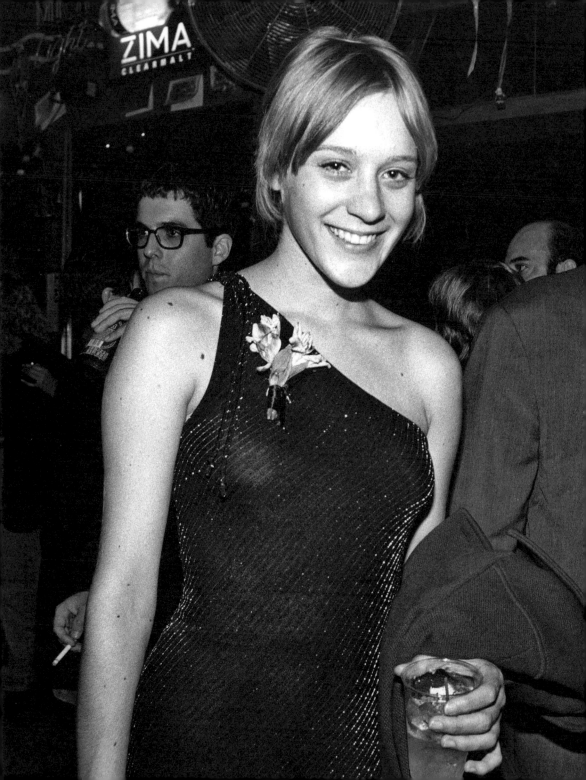

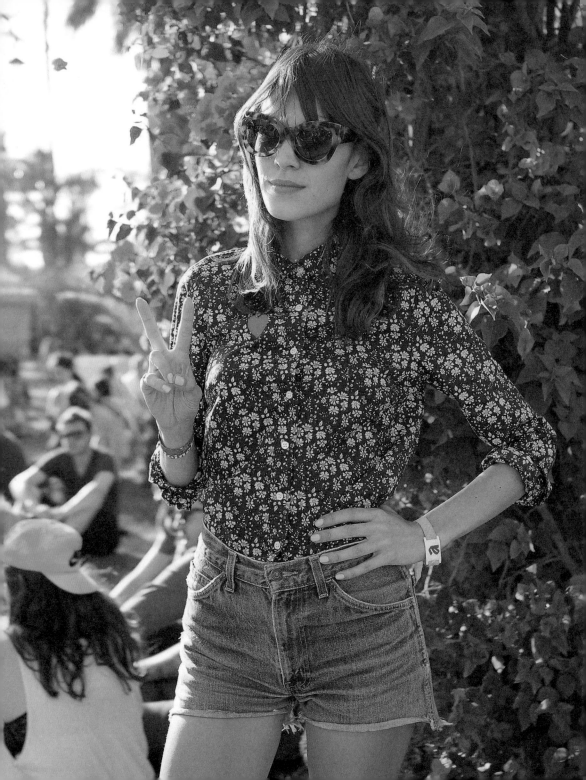

ALEXA CHUNG

UK, born 1983

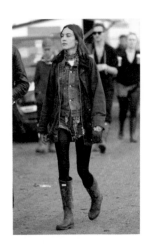

'Every time you post a picture of yourself to Instagram looking fake happy, a fairy dies.'

The thing about Alexa Chung is not that you necessarily want to be her friend, but that you want to have her wardrobe. All of it. You have a crush on her choppy hair, her green eyes, her long legs and her general ability to be the life and soul of the party at all times, but really, you'd be more than happy with a bin bag full of her hand-me-downs. You'd hope that in there you'd find a striped T-shirt or two, a slightly prim blouse (you really aren't fussy about a frayed hem or a missing button), a pair of princessy shoes and possibly even a cape.

Chung really has changed the way we look. She somehow distils the mood at any time and pours it into whatever she happens to be wearing that day. She's made it OK to wear shorts with wellies (she was first scouted at Reading Festival, so festival dressing is her specialist subject); to wear your mother's waxed Barbour jacket; and to rediscover Peter Pan collars and girly dresses, as well as dungarees, trench coats and leather jackets shrugged over a crisp shirt (such an Alexa look). She's put her stamp of approval on floppy fedoras, espadrilles and the 2.55 Chanel bag. Other classics that have been given the Alexa touch include the tuxedo jacket, ballet flats, ankle boots and – bless her – socks. Her style veers from boyish to feminine and sophisticated, but she has an indefinable cool factor that makes everything she wears just … right.

It's not surprising that Chung has had a bag named after her (smart move, Mulberry). She's also designed her own collection and written books about her style. She can't walk down the street without crashing the website of whichever bag brand she's carrying. She says she is inspired by everything from Jane Birkin's insouciance (see page 136) to David Hockney's striped sweater. Whatever she has, it seems we all want it. Now.

RIHANNA

Barbados, born 1988

*'Be a girl with a mind,
a bitch with an attitude,
a lady with class.'*

There's nothing Rihanna can't do. She's a singer, songwriter, businesswoman, beauty queen and Hollywood star. She's a diva in so many fields, it's hard to know where her career will take her next.

Rihanna's rise to stardom was meteoric. A year after being scouted performing with her schoolfriends' girl group at the age of 15, she had been signed by Jay Z, and she went on to become the youngest solo artist to achieve 14 Number 1 hits on the Billboard Hot 100, and one of the bestselling artists of all time. Now she's turning the world of fashion and beauty upside down, too.

Few music stars cross over into the world of high fashion with quite as much impact as Rihanna. She's appeared on the cover of magazines from *Vogue* to *i-D*, starred in Dior's Secret Garden campaign (2015) and been awarded Style Icon by the Council of Fashion Designers of America. Her passion for fashion and new designers is infectious. We love her in a mountain of tulle by the British designer Molly Goddard (see page 94). We love her in an imperial

yellow brocade robe by the Chinese couturier Guo Pei, with a train so huge it wouldn't fit in her limo, for the Met Gala in 2015 (we also loved the pizza memes the train inspired). We love her in head-to-toe white denim, or in a classic Prince of Wales trouser suit to meet President Macron of France.

And if that wasn't enough to inspire her legion Instagram followers (63.3 million of them at the time of writing), her own brand, Fenty, is taking over from conventional labels that have been around for decades. She launched Fenty Puma in 2016, and has since added beauty and underwear to her ever-expanding empire. Fenty Beauty offers 40 shades of foundation, because she wants to include everyone, while her lingerie sizes range from 32A to 42DD.

Rihanna is part of a new breed of social-media megabrands appealing to a younger generation who are more likely to watch her give a YouTube make-up tutorial than get beauty tips from *Vogue*. She's introduced a level of choice and diversity that the rest of the beauty industry is racing to imitate. Watch her go.

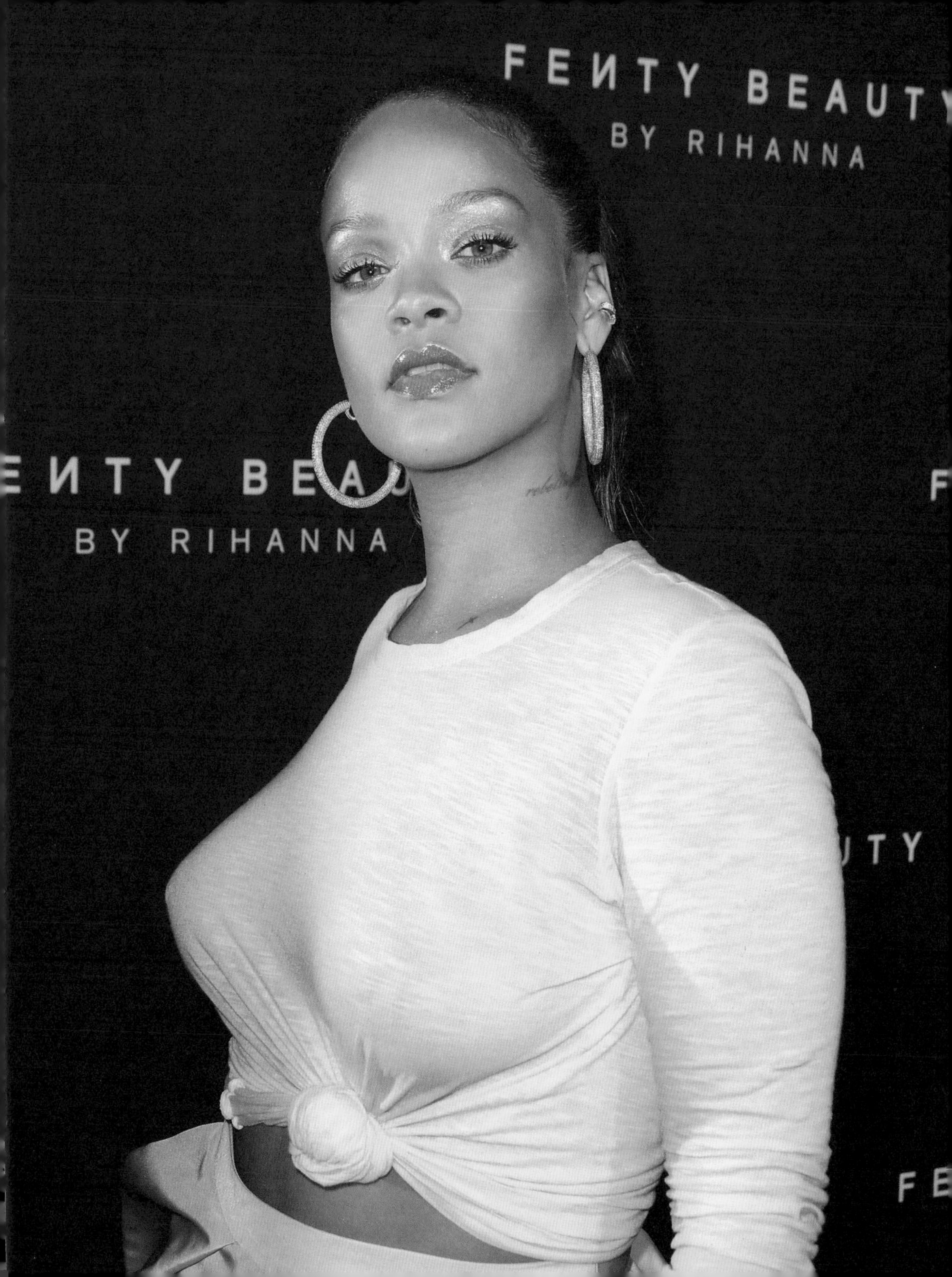
FENTY BEAUTY
BY RIHANNA
BY RIHANNA

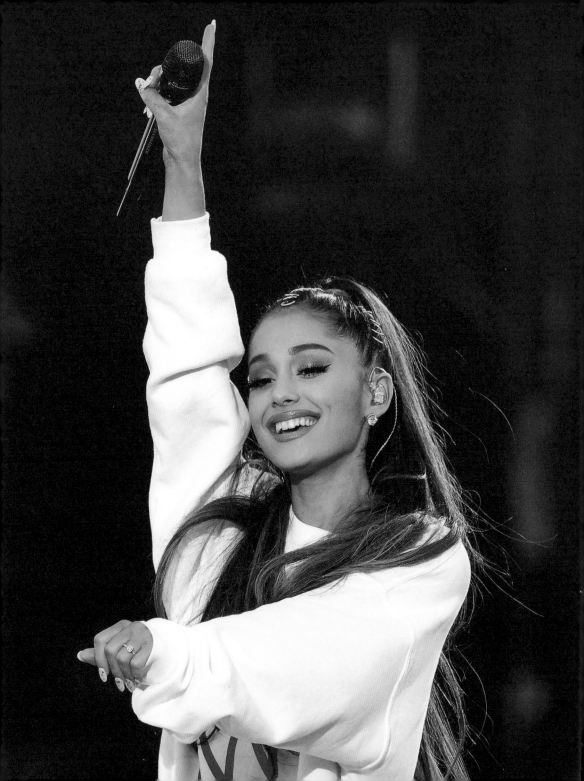

ARIANA GRANDE

USA, born 1993

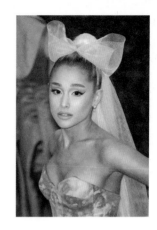

'We are not objects, we are QUEENS.'

With her high, scraped-back Barbie-doll ponytail, her tiny frame (1.5 m/less than 5 ft) in high shoes, her translucent complexion and her bouncy style, Ariana Grande is the ultimate bubblegum-pink pop princess. She's a phenomenon of the digital age, a Spotify star and a powerhouse on Instagram, with her own keyboard, Arimoji, and 131 million followers at the time of writing. On Twitter, she has more followers than most world leaders!

Born in Boca Raton, Florida, Grande burst on to television screens in 2010 at the age of 16 as Cat Valentine, a zany, red-haired singer wannabe in Nickelodeon's hit show *Victorious*, capturing the minds, hearts and imaginations of a generation of tweens. The transition from child star to grown-up was a rapid one, but she's been smart, mixing with all the right people, from obscure Norwegian DJs to Troye Sivan. And, of course, her friend Miley Cyrus.

Despite the lacy lingerie, shiny flasher rain mac, microskirt – or more likely no skirt at all – and thigh-high boots, Grande is also at the centre of a strong sisterhood, the Arianators. 'Misogyny is ever-present,'

she told *Coveteur* in 2017, 'and we have to be there to support one another. That's really it. It's about the sisterhood. There's no competing in that. We have to lift each other up, not try and claw each other down.' She is also a strong advocate for young LGBTQ kids, who feel drawn to the singer and her 'Break Free' message. She projects a strong feeling of love and positivity, and, since her One Love Manchester fund-raising concert in June 2017, has become something of a hero in the UK.

You can dissect any of Grande's looks and see her influence on mainstream fashion, not least the effect she has had on the athleisure range on which she collaborates with Reebok. If you're not comfortable in six-inch spike heels, a pair of Reebok Princess trainers will do just as well. Other trends she has spawned include brightly coloured plastic macs (she wore them before they were on Prada's catwalk), oversized sweatshirts, which have been adopted as the uniform of a generation along with bra tops, skinny black jeans, stonewash jeans and, of course, her trademark bunny ears, which became a symbol of solidarity after the terrorist attack following her concert in Manchester in May 2017.

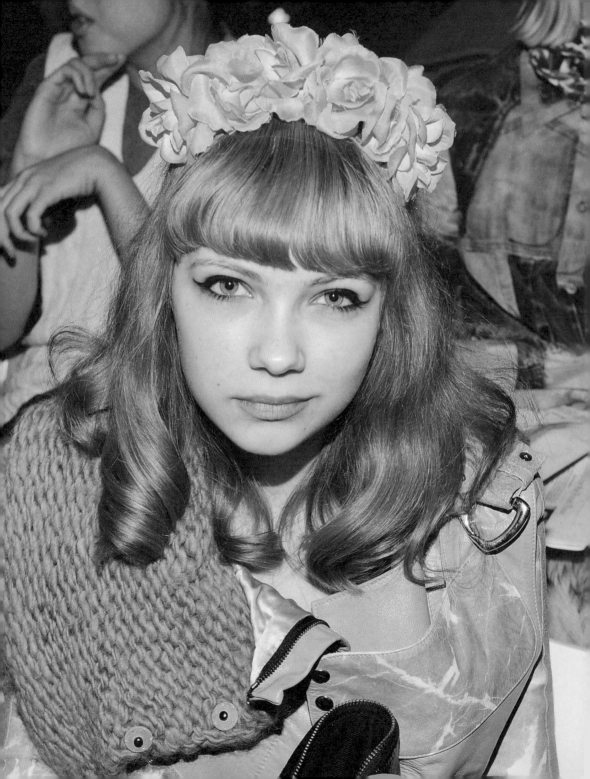

TAVI
GEVINSON

USA, born 1996

'Just be Stevie Nicks.
That's all you have to do.'

Anyone who remembers Tavi Gevinson's early days as a blogger – she started *Style Rookie* in 2008 – will feel as though they have grown up with her. She was just 11 years old, with an interest in fashion keener than most, and a sense of style so original – a kind of extraordinary Japanese anime granny-child with grey hair and specs – that fashion houses were shrinking their sizes so she could wear their pieces.

For a while, Gevinson was the girl crush of the entire fashion business, from Rei Kawakubo (see page 44) and Yohji Yamamoto to Karl Lagerfeld and Marc Jacobs. They invited her to their shows, and by the age of 13 she had done the front row, edited a 'zine for *Pop Magazine* in London and been flown to countless art and fashion openings.

Gevinson describes herself as a 'pop culture nerd'. It isn't just clothes; it's also music, books, art and, above all, film. She sucks it all up, a curious mind in an ever more curious world. By the time she was 15 her blog had evolved into an online magazine, *Rookie*, with a print spin-off in the form of an annual, *The Rookie Yearbook*. The power of a teenage girl with something to say – and a platform from which to say it – is awe-inspiring, and Gevinson made it seem that anything was possible. *Rookie* is still a thriving, inclusive community, addressing a different theme each month, from 'on the verge' to 'show and tell' and 'fear itself'.

At 18, Gevinson moved from her parents' house in suburban Chicago to actor's digs in downtown Chicago for her debut theatre run in *This Is our Youth*, by Kenneth Lonergan. She currently lives in New York and is an accomplished actor, speaker and writer. It feels as though she has already lived at least three lives, but with Gevinson, you know it is only the beginning.

IMAGE INFO

6 Aboah Adwoah, New York, 2017 (David X Prutting/BFA/REX/Shutterstock);

Fashion Plates

8 Lisa Fonssagrives, London,1951 by Toni Frissell (Library of Congress, Prints & Photographs Division, Toni Frissell Collection via Wikimedia Commons);

10 Lisa Fonssagrives photographed by Erwin Blumenfeld for French *Vogue*, Paris, 1939 (© The Estate of Erwin Blumenfeld);

11 Photographer Horst and Lisa Fonssagrives, 1949. (Photo by Roy Stevens/The LIFE Images Collection/Getty Images);

13 Dovima photographed by Erwin Blumenfeld for *Vogue*, August 1950 (© The Estate of Erwin Blumenfeld);

14 Twiggy, 1967 (Popperfoto/Getty Images);

16 Penelope Tree, London, 1967. Photograph by Patrick Lichfield (Lichfield/Getty Images);

17 Penelope Tree, New York, 1967 (Richard Swift/Penske Media/REX/Shutterstock);

18 Pat Cleveland, New York, 1977 (Chris Barham/Associated Newspapers/REX/Shutterstock);

20 Naomi Campbell for Azzedine Alaïa A/W 1992, Paris (Guy Marineau/Conde Nast via Getty Images);

22 Kate Moss photographed by Corinne Day for the cover of *The Face*, July 1990 (Courtesy Mix Mag Media, photo © Corinne Day/Trunk);

23 Kate Moss, London, 1993 (Richard Young/REX/Shutterstock);

24 Adwoa Aboah at the Gurls Talk Festival, 2018, New York (Cindy Ord/Getty Images);

25 Adwoa Aboah, Paris, 2017 (Cornel Cristian Petrus/REX/Shutterstock);

26 Cara Delevingne, London, 2017 (Jeff Spicer/Getty Images);

28 Gigi Hadid for Moschino A/W 2015, Milan (Pietro D'Aprano/Getty Images);

29 Gigi Hadid, New York, 2016 (Lars Niki/Corbis via Getty Images);

True Originals

30 Frida Kahlo, 1932 (Guillermo Kahlo via Wikimedia Commons);

32 Luisa Casati in a diamond-encrusted costume by Worth, Paris, 1922 (Hulton Archive/Getty Images);

33 Luisa Casati dressed as Queen Theodolinda, c.1905 (Archivio GBB/Contrasto/eyevine);

34 Georgia O'Keeffe photographed at her ranch in New Mexico by Philippe Halsman, 1948. (Philippe Halsman/Magnum Photos);

37 Diana Vreeland photographed in her living room by Horst P. Horst, New York, 1979 (Horst P Horst/Conde Nast via Getty Images);

38 Frida Kahlo, Mexico, 1932 (GL Archive/Alamy Stock Photo);

39 Frida Kahlo, Coyoacán, Mexico, 1948 (Bridgeman Images);

40 Anna Piaggi, London, 2006 (Chris Jackson/Getty Images);

42 Peggy Moffitt, Southampton, UK, 1965 (Mirrorpix/Alamy Stock Photo);

43 Peggy Moffitt models a dress for designer Rudi Gernreich, 1968 (Sal Traina/Penske Media/REX/Shutterstock);

45 Rei Kawakubo, Tokyo, 2005 (courtesy Eiichiro Sakata/Comme des Garçons);

46 Tina Chow with Tony Viramontes at Mr Chow, New York, c.1980 (Tony Viramontes Studio Archive);

47 Tina Chow, 1987 (Bernard Gotfryd/Getty Images);

48 Kate Bush, c.1970s (Peter Mazel/Sunshine/REX/Shutterstock);

49 Kate Bush, c.1985 (Kevin Cummins/Getty Images);

50 Madonna in *Desperately Seeking Susan*, 1985 (Herb Ritts/Orion Pictures/Kobal/REX/Shutterstock);

51 Madonna performs during her Blonde Ambition tour, Rotterdam, 1990 (Gie Knaeps/Getty Images);

52 Isabella Blow wears the lobster hat by milliner Philip Treacy, London, 1998 (Chris Moore/Catwalking);

53 Isabella Blow wears the Chinese garden headdress, created for Alexander McQueen S/S 2005 by Philip Treacy (Richard Saker/REX/Shutterstock);

54 Björk, Tokyo, 2016 (Santiago Felipe/Getty Images);

55 Björk, c.1990s (Jann Lipka/NordicPhotos/Alamy Stock Photo);

Punk Princesses

56 Courtney Love performs in Melbourne, 1995 (© Andrzej Liguz and moreimages.net via Wikimedia Commons);

58 Yoko Ono, New York, 1973 (Ron Galella/WireImage/Getty Images);

59 Yoko Ono, New York, 1974 (The Estate of David Gahr/Getty Images);

61 Vivienne Westwood, London, 2005 (Marc Larkin/LFI/Photoshot/Avalon.red);

62 Debbie Harry, London, 1978 (Brian Cooke/Redferns/Getty Images);

63 Debbie Harry, New York, 1977 (Waring Abbott/Michael Ochs Archives/Getty Images);

65 Marianne Faithfull by Michael Cooper, 1967 (© Michael Cooper Collection);

67 Patti Smith, Amsterdam, 1976 (Gijsbert Hanekroot/Redferns/Getty Images);

69 Poly Styrene, 1977 (Trinity Mirror/Mirrorpix/Alamy Stock Photo);

70 Ari Up performs with The Slits, London, 1977 (Ian Dickson/REX/Shutterstock);

71 Ari Up, California, 1980 (Hulton Archive/Getty Images);

72 Courtney Love in her apartment, 1995 (Kevin Cummins/Getty Images);

73 Courtney Love, LA, 1995 (Vinnie Zuffante/Getty Images);

74 Beth Ditto, Paris, 2010 (Dominique Charriau/WireImage/Getty Images);

Fashion Girlfriends

76 Leandra Medine, 2016 (Tradlands, CC BY 2.0, via Wikimedia Commons);

78 Coco Chanel in front of her home, Paris, 1929 (Sasha/Getty Images);

79 Coco Chanel, Paris, 1936 (Lipnitzki/Roger Viollet/Getty Images);

80 Elsa Schiaparelli wears a dress of her own design for American *Vogue*, September 1940 (Fredrich Baker/Condé Nast via Getty Images);

82 Claire McCardell, New York, 1940 (Bettmann/Getty Images);

83 Claire McCardell photographed by Erwin Blumenfeld, wearing her 'future dress', 1945 (© The Estate of Erwin Blumenfeld);

85 Mary Quant, London, 1966 (Giancarlo Botti/Gamma-Rapho via Getty Images);

86 Grace Coddington, 1967 (McKeown/Express/Hulton Archive/Getty Images);

87 Grace Coddington in her apartment, New York, 2016 (Clement Pascal/The New York Times/eyevine);

88 Donna Karan, New York, 1985 (James M Thresher/the Washington Post via Getty Images);

90 Miuccia Prada, Milan, 2009 (SPG/REX/Shutterstock);

92 Phoebe Philo at the finale of the Céline Ready-to-Wear A/W 2012 show, Paris, 2011 (Michel Dufour/WireImage/Getty Images);

93 Phoebe Philo, London, 2006 (Dave M Benet/Getty Images);

95 Molly Goddard, London, 2016 (Karwai Tang/WireImage/Getty Images);

96 Leandra Medine, New York, 2015 (Benjamin Lozovsky/BFA.com/REX/Shutterstock);

97 Leandra Medine, New York, 2016 (Daniel Zuchnik/Getty Images);

98 Kylie Jenner, New York, 2017 (Clint Spaulding/WWD/REX/Shutterstock);

99 'kyliejennershop.com' photo and website link posted on Instagram, 08/05/2017 (Private/Insight Media/Avalon.red);

Silver-Screen Dreams

100 Marlene Dietrich in *No Highway*, 1951 (20th Century Fox via Wikimedia Commons);

102 Marlene Dietrich in a publicity still for *Shanghai Express*, 1932 (William Walling/John Kobal Foundation/Getty Images);

103 Marlene Dietrich, LA, 1932 (Eugene Robert Richee/John Kobal Foundation/Getty Images);

104 Greta Garbo in *A Woman of Affairs*, 1928 (MGM/Bettmann/Getty Images);

107 Katharine Hepburn photographed for *LIFE* magazine by Alfred Eisenstaedt, New York, 1938 (Alfred Eisenstaedt/The LIFE Images Collection/Getty Images);

108 Rita Hayworth, 1941 (John Kobal Foundation/Getty Images);

109 Rita Hayworth in *Gilda*, 1946 (Columbia/George Rinhart/Corbis via Getty Images);

111 Lauren Bacall in a publicity still for *The Big Sleep*, 1946 (Sunset Boulevard/Corbis via Getty Images);

112 Marilyn Monroe in *Some Like It Hot*, 1959 (United Artists/Diltz/Bridgeman Images);

113 Marilyn Monroe photographed by Alfred Eisenstaedt for *LIFE* magazine, LA, May 1953 (Alfred Eisenstaedt/The LIFE Images Collection/Getty Images);

114 Diane Keaton, LA, 1973 (Rosen Allen/Penske Media/REX/Shutterstock);

116 Tilda Swinton, Cannes, 2013 (Matt Baron/BEI/REX/Shutterstock);

118 Lupita Nyong'o at the 86th Academy Awards, LA, 2014 (Stewart Cook/REX/Shutterstock);

119 Lupita Nyong'o, London, 2016 (Karwai Tang/WireImage/Getty Images);

The It Girls

120 Audrey Hepburn, 1954 (Hans Gerber/ETH Bibliothek Zürich, Bildarchiv/Com_X-H061-013 /CC BY-SA 4.0 via Wikimedia);

122 Audrey Hepburn at a fitting with Hubert de Givenchy, c.1950s (Screen Prod/Photononstop/Alamy Stock Photo);

123 Audrey Hepburn, 1952 (Archive Photos/Getty Images);

124 Brigitte Bardot, Cannes, 1953 (Sipa Press/REX/Shutterstock);

126 Jean Seberg in *Breathless*, 1960 (Les Films Impéria/Photoshot/Avalon.red);

127 Jean Seberg and Jean-Paul Belmondo in *Breathless*, 1960 (Les Films Impéria/Photoshot/Avalon.red);

129 Edie Sedgwick photographed by Frederick Eberstadt for *LIFE* magazine, November 1965 (© Frederick Eberstadt);

130 Catherine Deneuve, c.1962 (Silver Screen Collection/Getty Images);

131 Catherine Deneuve with Yves Saint Laurent, Paris, 1966 (David Raymond/Library/REX/Shutterstock);

132 Françoise Hardy, 1965 (Michael Ochs Archives/Getty Images);

133 Françoise Hardy, 1969 (Reg Lancaster/Express/Getty Images);

134 Vidal Sassoon cuts Mia Farrow's hair in a promotion for *Rosemary's Baby*, 1967 (Max B Miller/Fotos International/Getty Images);

136 Jane Birkin and Serge Gainsbourg, Paris, 1969 (Keystone-France/Gamma-Keystone via Getty Images);

137 Jane Birkin, 1974 (A Di Crollalanza/REX/Shutterstock);

139 Jeny Howorth walks for Claude Montana S/S 1987 (Daniel Simon/Gamma-Rapho via Getty Images);

141 Winona Ryder, LA, 1989 (Ron Galella/WireImage/Getty Images);

Pioneers

142 Amelia Earhart c 1928. (Library of Congress, Prints & Photographs Division, Underwood & Underwood via Wikimedia Commons);

144 Amelia Earhart photographed by Edward Steichen for *Vanity Fair*, 1931 (Edward Steichen/Condé Nast via Getty Images);

145 Amelia Earhart, New Jersey, 1932 (© SZ Photo/Scherl/Bridgeman Images);

147 Josephine Baker, Paris, 1931 (Roger-Viollet/REX/Shutterstock);

148 Lee Miller, *Self Portrait with Head Band*, New York, c.1932 (© Lee Miller Archives, England 2018. All rights reserved. leemiller.co.uk);

149 Lee Miller in uniform at the Vogue studios, London, 1943 (David E Scherman © Courtesy Lee Miller Archives, England 2018. All rights reserved);

151 Billie Holiday performs on stage, 1950 (Gilles Petard/Redferns/Getty Images);

152 Margaret Thatcher interviewed by *L'Express* in January, London, 1988 (Jean Guichard/Gamma-Rapho via Getty Images);

154 Gloria Steinem, New York, 1970 (*NY Daily News* via Getty Images);

155 Gloria Steinem appears in *LIFE* magazine, August 1965 (Yale Joel/The LIFE Images Collection/Getty Images);

157 Prime Minister Margaret Thatcher greets Katharine Hamnett at 10 Downing Street, London, 1984 (PA Images);

158 Anna Wintour, New York, 2014 (Leandro Justen/BFANYC.com/REX/Shutterstock);

159 Anna Wintour, Milan, 2015 (Comi/Terenghi/REX/Shutterstock);

161 Stella McCartney at the finale of the Stella McCartney S/S 2017 show, Paris, 2016 (Estrop/Getty Images);

162 Elaine Welteroth, New York, 2017 (Billy Farrell/BFA/REX/Shutterstock);

163 Elaine Welteroth, New York, 2018 (Pixelformula/SIPA/REX/Shutterstock);

Cleopatras

164 Elizabeth Taylor, c 1955 (20th Century Fox/doctormacro.com via Wikimedia Commons);

166 Theda Bara in *Cleopatra*, 1917 (Silver Screen Collection/Getty Images);

168 Elizabeth Taylor in *Cleopatra*, 1963 (20th Century Fox/LFI/Photoshot/Avalon.red);

169 Elizabeth Taylor, 1955 (Silver Screen Collection/Getty Images);

170 Nina Simone performs at the Newport Jazz Festival, Rhode Island, 1968 (David Redfern/Redferns/Getty Images);

172 The Ronettes perform in 1965 (Michael Ochs Archives/Getty Images);

173 Ronnie Spector, 1964 (Michael Ochs Archives/Getty Images);

174 Siouxsie Sioux, 1979 (Fin Costello/Redferns/Getty Images);

175 Siouxsie Sioux performs in London, 1978 (Gus Stewart/Redferns/Getty Images);

176 Tracey Emin, 2000 (Idols/Photoshot/Avalon.red);

178 Christian Dior S/S 2004 Haute Couture, Paris (LFI/Photoshot/Avalon.red);

179 Pat McGrath with Natalia Vodianova, backstage at Calvin Klein S/S 2006 (Retna/Photoshot/Avalon.red);

180 Amy Winehouse performs at the MTV Movie Awards, LA, 2007 (Jeff Kravitz/FilmMagic/Getty Images);

Blue Bloods

182 Grace Kelly in *The Country Girl*, 1954 (Paramount via Wikimedia Commons);

185 Duchess of Windsor, 1940 (THE LIFE Images Collection/Getty Images);

186 Mona Williams, later Mona von Bismarck, photographed by Cecil Beaton for *Vogue*, February 1948 (Cecil Beaton/Condé Nast via Getty Images);

187 Mona Williams, date unknown (Bettmann/Getty Images);

189 Deborah Mitford, High Wycombe, UK, 1940 (Central Press/Hulton Archive/Getty Images);

190 Gloria Vanderbilt photographed at home by Horst P. Horst for US *Vogue*, April 1966 (Horst P Horst/Conde Nast via Getty Images);

192 Jacqueline Kennedy Onassis, Capri, 1971 (Rolls Press/Popperfoto/Getty Images);

193 Jacqueline Kennedy, then First Lady of the United States, India, 1962 (Art Rickerby/The LIFE Picture Collection/Getty Images);

194 Grace Kelly on horseback on the set of a film, probably *Mogambo*, 1953 (Gene Lester/Getty Images);

195 Grace Kelly photographed by Philippe Halsman in the gown she wore to the 27th Academy Awards, 1955 (Philippe Halsman/Magnum Photos);

196 Diane von Furstenberg, 1973 (ADC/REX/Shutterstock);

199 Inès de la Fressange models Chanel spring fashions, c.1980s (Michel Arnaud/Corbis via Getty Images);

200 Princess Diana arrives at the Serpentine, London, 1994 (Nils Jorgensen/REX/Shutterstock);

201 Princess Diana, London, 1982 (Anwar Hussein/WireImage/Getty Images);

202 Stella Tennant, 1990 (The LIFE Images Collection/Getty Images);

203 Stella Tennant for Chanel A/W 2011, Paris (REX/Shutterstock);

205 Meghan, Duchess of Sussex, Windsor, UK, 2018 (Anwar Hussein/Getty Images);

Girl Crushes

206 Sofia Coppola, Cannes, 2013 (Georges Biard, CC BY-SA 3.0, from Wikimedia Commons);

208 Cyndi Lauper, 1980 (Barry King/WireImage/Getty Images);

210 Sade Adu, 1986 (Peter Jordan/The LIFE Images Collection/Getty Images);

211 Sade Adu, 1980 (David Montgomery/Getty Images);

212 Neneh Cherry, c.1980s (Travis Watson);

214 Molly Ringwald, LA, 1985 (Bob Riha Jr/Getty Images);

215 Molly Ringwald, 1983 (Sipa Press/REX/Shutterstock);

216 Sofia Coppola, Rome, 2013 (Davide Lanzilao/Contrasto/eyevine);

218 Chloë Sevigny, Utah, 2016 (Stephen Lovekin/Variety/REX/Shutterstock);

219 Chloë Sevigny, New York, 1996 (Catherine McGann/Getty Images);

220 Alexa Chung at Coachella Music Festival, California, 2013 (David X Prutting/BFAnyc.com/REX/Shutterstock);

221 Alexa Chung at Glastonbury, UK, 2015 (David Sims/ WENN.com);

223 Rihanna, New York, 2017 (Matt Baron/REX/Shutterstock);

224 Ariana Grande performs at the One Love Manchester benefit concert, UK, 2017 (Getty Images/Dave Hogan for One Love Manchester);

225 Ariana Grande, New York, 2018 (Startraks Photo/REX/Shutterstock);

226 Tavi Gevinson, New York, 2012 (Jesse Lirola/BFA/REX/Shutterstock).

INDEX

ACKNOWLEDGMENTS

This is to thank all the women I have admired, crushed on and fan-girled over through the years, particularly Lauren Bacall, Marilyn, Madonna, Billie Holiday and Katharine Hamnett.

Thank you Mark, for sharing the load and being so supportive, Fred, for always taking an interest, and Sybilla, for showing me the next generation of women who are changing the way we look. Special thanks to Megan Doyle and a lifetime's supply of Violet's buns to Kathryn Holliday.

With grateful thanks to Katherine Pitt for her patience and calm editing, Mariana Sameiro for designing such a beautiful book, Giulia Hetherington for her comprehensive picture research and Camilla Morton, without whom this book would not have happened.

Most of all, in loving memory of Min, who truly shaped the way I look.